DC:0-3R

Diagnostic Classification of
Mental Health and
Developmental Disorders of
Infancy and Early Childhood
REVISED EDITION

The DC:0–3R Revision Task Force

Helen Link Egger

Emily Fenichel

Antoine Guedeney

Brian K. Wise

Harry H. Wright

Robert N. Emde, Chair

DC:0–3R

Diagnostic Classification of
Mental Health and
Developmental Disorders of
Infancy and Early Childhood
REVISED EDITION

ZERO TO THREE

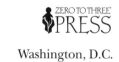

Washington, D.C.

Published by

ZERO TO THREE
2000 M St., NW, Suite 200
Washington, DC 20036-3307
(202) 638-1144
Toll-free orders (800) 899-4301
Fax: (202) 638-0851
Web: http://www.zerotothree.org

Cover design: Kelly Rozwadowski, K Art and Design
Text design and composition: Seven Worldwide Publishing Solutions

Library of Congress Cataloging-in-Publication Data

Diagnostic classification, 0-3.
  Diagnostic classification of mental health and developmental disorders of infancy
and early childhood : DC:0-3R.– Rev.
      p. cm.
  Rev. ed. of: Diagnostic classification, 0-3.
  ISBN 0-943657-90-3
  1. Child psychopathology–Classification. 2. Infant psychiatry–Classification.
3. Child psychopathology–Diagnosis. 4. Infant psychiatry–Diagnosis. 5. Child
psychopathology–Case studies. 6. Infant psychiatry–Case studies. I. Title: DC:0-3R.
II. Zero to Three (Organization). III. Title.
  RJ500.5.D53 2005
  618.92'89'0012–dc22
                           2005015438

10 9 8 7 6 5 4 3 2 1
ISBN-13: 978-0-943657-90-5
ISBN-10: 0-943657-90-3
Printed in the United States of America

Suggested citation:
ZERO TO THREE. (2005). *Diagnostic classification of mental health and developmental
disorders of infancy and early childhood: Revised edition (DC:0–3R)*. Washington, DC.
ZERO TO THREE Press.

Table of Contents

Acknowledgments

The Revision Task Force acknowledges with thanks the help given us by the global community of infant mental health clinicians and researchers who responded to our requests for information and feedback about DC:0–3 during the many phases of our review process. Ten years after the publication of DC:0–3, hundreds of individuals and a number of groups gave us useful advice that reflected the fruits of a decade of experience. These hundreds of respondents are clearly committed to advancing clinical work with very young children and their families by updating diagnostic classification by means of specifying criteria that are based on current knowledge and evidence. This community's expressed compassion for vulnerable infants, toddlers, and their families everywhere gives us hope for the future.

Special thanks are due to those who reported clinical trials of DC:0–3 and contributed to the recent literature on diagnostic classification in early childhood. Following the traditions of diagnostic classification guides, we have not cited references for the vast majority of contributions that we reviewed. A future publication will provide an overview of citations and our evaluation of the much-appreciated evidence that backs up our revision.

We are grateful to everyone who responded to the Revision Task Force's two surveys in 2003. Respondents included practicing clinicians from a range of disciplines, as well as those engaged in research and administration in the infant mental health field.

A number of groups provided crucial information or feedback that guided our efforts. A group of occupational therapists, chaired by Lucy Miller, guided our work on Regulation Disorders of Sensory Processing. A group of clinicians experienced with Posttraumatic Stress Disorder, chaired by Neil Boris, helped to shape our efforts on that classification. Robert Harmon and Jean Thomas provided guidance from the perspective of training practitioners in the use of DC:0–3. An independent working group, chaired by Michael Scheeringa and generously supported by the American Academy of Child and Adolescent Psychiatry (AACAP), developed the Research Diagnostic Criteria, Preschool Age (RDC-PA Task Force on Research Diagnostic Criteria: Infancy and Preschool, 2003) subsequently published by AACAP, that informed our approach and contributed substantially to a number of criteria that are included in DC:0–3R. We are grateful for the evidence-based work of this group that allows us to link our classification system to the preschool ages. As documented in our introduction, two members of the DC:0–3R Revision Task Force had been members of the RDC-PA group.

A number of individuals deserve special acknowledgment for their constructive contributions at key points. Serena Wieder provided her perspectives for disorders of regulation and Axis V as well as her views on the role of classification in general. Catherine Lord, Roseanne Clark, Thomas Anders, and Charles Zeanah generously shared their expertise.

As we moved closer to the final version of our revision, several experts agreed to review our document and offer detailed suggestions. We are grateful to Arnold Sameroff, Jean Thomas, Alice Carter, Joy Osofsky, and Alicia Lieberman for serving in this role.

Without the encouragement of ZERO TO THREE, its Executive Director, Matthew Melmed, and its Executive Committee, the creation of DC:0–3R would never have been accomplished. We are also grateful for the superb staff support for our work provided by Margaret Henry and Crystal Wiggins, who gave continued attention to details and coordinated our efforts.

Finally, we owe a huge debt of gratitude to the original task group that constructed DC:0–3. The members of this group, chaired by Stanley Greenspan and Serena Wieder, are fully acknowledged in Appendix C. DC:0–3R goes forward because of their pioneering work.

The Revision Task Force

Helen Link Egger
Emily Fenichel
Antoine Guedeney
Brian K. Wise
Harry H. Wright

Robert N. Emde, Chair

Introduction

ZERO TO THREE's *Diagnostic Classification of Mental Health and Developmental Disorders of Infancy and Early Childhood* (DC:0–3), published in 1994, was designed to address the need for a systematic, developmentally based approach to the classification of mental health and developmental difficulties in the first 4 years of life. The creation of DC:0–3 represented the first-ever attempt by a group of experienced clinicians to formulate a useful scheme that would complement, but not replace, existing medical and developmental frameworks such as *The Diagnostic and Statistical Manual of Mental Disorders of the American Psychiatric Association* (DSM-III-R, 1987); and the *International Classification of Diseases* of the World Health Organization (ICD 9). The developers of DC:0–3 sought to take account of new knowledge concerning (1) factors that contribute to adaptive and maladaptive patterns of development and (2) the meaning of individual differences in infancy. Their goal was to provide classification criteria that could advance professional communication, as well as clinical formulation and research. This manual, developed a decade after the publication of the original classification system, provides a revision that updates criteria for classifications, incorporates new knowledge from clinical experience, and attempts to clarify areas of persistent ambiguity.

The Origins of DC:0–3

DC:0–3 was the product of a multidisciplinary Diagnostic Classification Task Force that was established in 1987 by ZERO TO THREE: National Center for Infants, Toddlers, and Families, an organization representing interdisciplinary professional leadership in the field of infant development and mental health. Task force members included clinicians and researchers from infant mental health centers throughout North America and Europe. Members of the group systematically analyzed case reports from participating centers, identified recurring patterns of behavioral problems, and described categories of disorders. The process was an open one, in which opinions were sought from a variety of disciplines.

Through expert consensus, an initial set of diagnostic categories emerged. Task Force members recognized that, given the limitations of infant mental health knowledge, diagnostic categories in the new classification system could only be descriptive—that is, representative of meaningful symptom patterns. Sometimes categorical descriptions included associated events (e.g., between a traumatic event and a group of symptoms) or developmental features (e.g., between sensory or motor patterns and a group of symptoms seen at a particular stage of early development). The result was a scheme based on five axes:

- Axis I: Primary Diagnosis
- Axis II: Relationship Disorder Classification
- Axis III: Medical and Developmental Disorders and Conditions
- Axis IV: Psychosocial Stressors
- Axis V: Functional Emotional Developmental Level

Having accomplished this, the Task Force recognized that this new guide for diagnostic classification of mental disorders in this age group would be tentative. Wording from the Introduction to DC:0–3 is instructive.

> In any scientific enterprise, but particularly in a new field, a healthy tension exists between the desire to analyze findings from systematic research before offering even initial conceptualizations and the need to disseminate preliminary conceptualizations so that they can serve as a basis for collecting systematic data, which can lead to more empirically based efforts. . . . . The development of DC:0–3 represents an important first step: the presentation of expert, consensus-based categorizations of mental health and developmental disorders in the early years of life. . . . . It is an initial guide for clinicians and researchers to facilitate clinical diagnosis and planning, as well as communication and further research (p. 11).

The Usefulness of DC:0–3 and the Need for Revision

Clinicians who address the mental health needs of infants and young children welcomed DC:0–3 and found it useful for clinical formulation. Translations of DC:0–3 have been published in Dutch, French, German, Italian, Korean, Portuguese, Serbian, and Spanish. Limited-circulation translations have been made in additional languages.

Considering its wide usage, one might ask, Why the need for revision of DC:0–3? There are several reasons. First, any diagnostic classification system, especially a new one, should be reviewed and updated a decade after publication. The developers of DC:0–3 intended the system to evolve. Second, and more specifically, users over the years have pointed out limitations in the usefulness of DC:0–3's criteria. Some classification categories lacked criteria altogether; other categories had criteria that required clarification. Criteria that were stated in general terms in DC:0–3 required more specific "operational" language in order to be useful for communication and research. Third, as increasing numbers of clinicians were finding DC:0–3 valuable not only for communicating about disorders but also for clinical formulation of individual cases and treatment planning (see section below on the diagnostic process and clinical formulation), the system required review from that perspective. Equally important, a revision of DC:0–3 provided an opportunity to incorporate new knowledge and clinical experience into this resource for early childhood mental health.

In contemplating a revision of DC:0–3, the continuing developers of the system recognized that most clinicians would expect a revision to include data from evaluation of the system. The evaluation of any diagnostic classification system should include its coverage of clinical syndromes and problems, as well as its overall usefulness in terms of practice, training, and research. Clinical trials are essential to establish the reliability and validity of a system. Not surprisingly, considering the lack of specificity of DC:0–3's criteria, the clinical trials of DC:0–3 that were reported in the literature in the decade following its publication had scant or no information concerning clinicians' ability to make reliable judgments about classification. The Special Issue of the *Infant Mental Health Journal* devoted to trials of DC:0–3 is illustrative (Guedeney & Maestro, 2003). Summaries of trials conducted in Montreal, Tel-Aviv, Paris, Lisbon, and Topeka suggested that the first three axes of DC:0–3 were useful in classifying disorders and that the coverage of disorders reflected the span of cases seen at different referral sites. DC:0–3 was also found useful in clinical formulation. However, the fact that researchers reported reliability in only two of these five trials indicated the need for more attention to this area.

If a classification system is to survive, let alone evolve and be used in research, its validity needs to be established by means of links to other recognized assessments and to outcomes over time. But, as researchers observe, reliability sets the upper limit on assessments of validity. Clarity of communication depends in large measure on the degree to which clinicians can agree on a diagnostic classification when they see the same data about a patient. It is only when regularly agreed-upon units are established and the extent of agreement about these units is known that researchers can go on to evaluate a classification system's link to other assessments and patient outcomes. Thus, although a growing number of clinicians, educators, and developers of early childhood mental health systems of care were finding DC:0–3 useful, especially in comparison to other classification systems, the developers of DC:0–3 recognized the need to revise its criteria in order to promote reliability. Only then could clinical trials foster the continued evolution of DC:0–3.

After reviewing the five clinical trials of DC:0–3 and issues of reliability and validity, Emde and Wise (2003) proposed that ZERO TO THREE undertake a circumscribed revision of the system. Such a revision would not change classification categories (unless there was a strong empirical reason to do so) but, rather, provide needed specifications and clarifications of criteria in order to facilitate reliability among clinicians and advance the evidence-based evolution of the system. In addition, a revision of DC:0–3 would be designed to improve its usefulness in clinical case formulation.

In late 2003, ZERO TO THREE appointed a Revision Task Force to draft a revised version of DC:0–3 within 2 years. The group reviewed clinical literature and other diagnostic systems, carried out two surveys of users worldwide, and obtained draft language and feedback from recognized experts in particular areas. The group conferred weekly, meeting via conference calls and in person in order to clarify text and diagnostic criteria. DC:0–3R is the product of this 2-year effort. (Details of the process of revision are presented in Appendix B.)

DC:0–3R in Relation to Other Classification Systems

DC:0–3 was intended to complement existing approaches to diagnostic classification of mental health and developmental disorders of infancy and early childhood. DC:0–3R continues this intention. DC:0–3 responded to the failure of the DSM system to include (1) sufficient coverage of syndromes of early childhood that needed clinical attention or (2) sufficient consideration of developmental features of early disorders. Interestingly, in the years since the publication of DC:0–3 (i.e., 0 *to* 3), clinicians have been using the system for the classification of disorders in the first 4 years (i.e., 0 *through* 3), with many finding the DC:0–3 system to be useful well into the preschool age period. This pattern of usage has resulted in a clear need to integrate DC:0–3R with DSM-IV (American Psychiatric Association, 1994) criteria for older children.

In 2001–2002, The American Academy of Child and Adolescent Psychiatry supported an independent work group that developed *Research Diagnostic Criteria-Preschool Age* (RDC-PA; Task Force on Research Diagnostic Criteria: Infancy and Preschool, 2003), which specifies psychiatric criteria for disorders seen among preschoolers. We have sought to incorporate these criteria into DC:0–3R wherever possible. It is important to note, however, the different goals of RDC-PA and DC:0–3 R. These can be summarized as follows:

- RDC-PA took *The Diagnostic and Statistical Manual of Mental Disorders, Fourth Edition, Text Revision* (DSM-IV-TR; American Psychiatric Association, 2000) classification categories as its point of departure and then specified developmentally appropriate criteria for preschoolers. In contrast, DC:0–3 and DC:0–3R include classification categories that have not been covered in the DSM system.

- RDC-PA focuses sharply on research diagnostic criteria, without considering clinical formulation or usefulness. DC:0–3 and DC:0–3R give central consideration to the latter features, including assessment of caregiving relationships and socio-emotional functioning.

- RDC-PA gives primary attention to the preschool period. DC:0–3 and DC:0–3R devote attention primarily to the first 3 years.

These differences notwithstanding, the congruence between RDC-PA and DC:0–3R is substantial. After reviewing new evidence for DSM-IV-TR–related classifications, the DC:0–3R Revision Task Force adopted the following classifications from RDC-PA:

- Subclassifications of anxiety disorder after the age of 2 years;

- The use of Pervasive Developmental Disorders (e.g. autism, PDD, NOS) after 2 years of age. (DC:0–3R retains Multisystem Developmental Disorder [MSDD] as a possible classification for children under the age of 2 years.);

- Subclassifications for Sleep Behavior Disorders; and

- Subclassifications for Feeding Behavior Disorders.

As was the case in DC:0–3, DC:0–3R encourages readers to refer to the DSM-IV-TR and the *International Classification of Diseases* of the World Health Organization (ICD 10; 1992), both of which describe a number of mental health disorders that are typically first diagnosed in infancy and early childhood. If a DSM-IV-TR diagnosis best describes the primary presenting difficulty, it should be coded under Axis I of DC:0–3R. For example, if the diagnosis is Pica, Rumination Disorder, or Obsessive-Compulsive Disorder—diagnoses that are not included in the DC:0–3 or DC:0–3R system—then the clinician should list the appropriate DSM-IV-TR diagnosis as the clinical disorder under Axis I of DC:0–3R. Similarly, if a preschooler presents evidence of an early disruptive behavior disorder—for example, Attention-Deficit Hyperactivity Disorder, Conduct Disorder, or Oppositional Defiant Disorder—the clinician may use the criteria of DSM-IV-TR, as adapted by RDC-PA (2003) for diagnostic classification. These disorders can be listed in Axis I under "Other Disorders (DSM-IV-TR or ICD 10)."

Many medical conditions and diseases of infancy and early childhood influence development in general and emotional development in particular. Such relevant medical conditions, described in classification frameworks such as ICD 10, should be listed under Axis III of DC:0–3R. Early childhood educators, speech/language pathologists, occupational therapists, and physical therapists use specialized classification frameworks to organize and systematize developmental findings related to communication, motor development, and sensory functioning. These diagnoses should also be listed under Axis III of DC:0–3R.

The Diagnostic Process and Clinical Formulation

Before proceeding to an overview of changes in DC:0–3R and remaining issues in its use, it seems appropriate to review some features of the diagnostic process in general, as well as some thoughts about clinical formulations in the context of early development.

The Diagnostic Process

For the practicing clinician, the diagnostic process is ongoing. One does not make a diagnosis on the basis of a onetime "snapshot" of symptoms, but rather one collects information over time in order to understand multiple aspects of presenting problems as well as variations in adaptation and development that reveal themselves on different occasions and in different contexts.

The diagnostic process consists of two aspects: the classification of disorders and the assessment of individuals. We classify disorders, not individuals. We classify disorders primarily so that professionals can communicate clearly about descriptive syndromes. Clinicians can then link their observations to a growing body of knowledge concerning etiology, pathogenesis, the course of a disorder, and expectations concerning treatment. Using the common language of a diagnostic classification system facilitates the connection of individuals to existing services and thus can aid in the mobilization of appropriate systems of mental health care. The assessment of individuals, however, necessarily precedes classification. Assessment and classification are both used in clinical formulation.

Clinical formulation involves the drawing together of multiple observations and sources of information about the individual within a general diagnostic scheme, so as to guide the clinician about what to do next. It is noteworthy that as DSM and ICD classification systems have evolved to be multiaxial, clinicians have used them not only for classification of disorders but also as guides for assessment and clinical formulation. The first three axes of these systems deal with the classification of disorders, and the fourth and fifth axes deal with the assessment of individuals in context. DC:0–3 and DC:0–3R follow a similar multiaxial scheme. DC:0–3R Axes I (Clinical Disorders), II (Relationship Classification), and III (Medical and Developmental Disorders and Conditions) deal with the classification of disorders. Axis IV (Psychosocial Stressors) and V (Emotional and Social Functioning) reflect the assessment of individuals in context.

Clinical Formulation in Infancy and Early Childhood

In discussing clinical formulation with respect to infants, toddlers, and young children, the authors of DC:0–3 made two key observations:

- Assessment and diagnostic classification are guided by the awareness that all infants have their own developmental progression and show individual differences in their motor, sensory, language, cognitive, affective, and interactive patterns.
- All infants and young children are participants in relationships. Children's most significant relationships are usually those within the family. Families, in turn, participate in relationships within their larger communities and cultures.

Any intervention or treatment program should be based on as complete an understanding of the child and the child's relationships as it is possible to achieve. Pressed for time, clinicians may be tempted to focus attention on a limited number of variables while giving only cursory regard to other influences on development. Clinicians may also be tempted to avoid assessing those areas of a child's functioning where the constructs or research tools are not fully developed or where gaps in their own training exist. Although these temptations are understandable, any clinician who is responsible for making a complete diagnostic assessment of an infant or young child and planning an appropriate intervention program must take into account all relevant areas of the child's functioning. Independently or with a team of colleagues, the clinician is obliged to apply state-of-the-art knowledge to each area of functioning and to evaluate both strengths and weaknesses in the child and family.

A clinician or team needs a number of sessions to understand how an infant, toddler, or young child is developing in each area of functioning. A few questions to parents or caregivers about each area may be appropriate for screening, but not for a full evaluation. A full evaluation usually requires a minimum of three to five sessions of 45 or more minutes each. A complete evaluation will typically involve:

- Interviewing the parent(s) about the child's developmental history;
- Direct observation of family functioning—for example, family and parental dynamics, the caregiver–child relationship, and interaction patterns;
- Gaining information, through direct observation and report, about the child's individual characteristics, language, cognition, and affective expression; and
- Assessment of sensory reactivity and processing, motor tone, and motor planning capacities.

In addition to consideration of clinical disorders, findings from a comprehensive evaluation should lead to preliminary notions about:

- The nature of the child's pattern of strengths and difficulties, including the level of overall adaptive capacity and functioning in the major areas of development (i.e., social–emotional, relational, cognitive, language, sensory, and motor abilities) in comparison to age-expected developmental patterns.
- The relative contribution to the child's competencies and difficulties of the different areas assessed (e.g., family relationships, interactive patterns, stress, and constitutional–maturational patterns).
- A comprehensive treatment or preventive intervention plan to deal with 1 and 2 above.

Provided that well-trained clinicians have sufficient time and resources to conduct them, comprehensive diagnostic assessments may take place in many different settings. A clinician who conducts a diagnostic evaluation and formulates an intervention plan should have experience in assessing the areas of functioning described above and in integrating the assessment findings into a cohesive formulation. Settings that are strong in only some areas of assessment and intervention should obtain additional expertise through engaging additional staff or through consultation with colleagues who have the expertise to assess specific areas of functioning. For example, the assessment of regulation disorders of sensory processing may require the expertise of an occupational therapist who is trained to evaluate sensory processing and integration capacities in infants and young children.

DC:0–3R continues the multiaxial classification system that has been so useful in clinical formulation. Use of the multiaxial system for clinical formulation focuses the clinician's attention on the factors that may be contributing to the difficulties of the infant or young child, adaptive strengths, and additional areas of functioning in which intervention may be needed. The labels for DC:0–3R's axes are essentially the same as those in DC:0–3, incorporating some changes in wording recommended by users. They are:

Axis I: Clinical Disorders

Axis II: Relationship Classification

Axis III: Medical and Developmental Disorders and Conditions

Axis IV: Psychosocial Stressors

Axis V: Emotional and Social Functioning

Each axis is described in detail in the pages that follow. Appendix A provides guidelines for thinking about diagnosis and selecting classifications.

A Summary of Changes in DC:0–3R

Most of the differences that distinguish DC:0–3R from DC:0–3 specify and clarify criteria for the classification categories already designated in Axis I of DC:0–3. Although the Revision Task Force did not intend to change or add major classification categories in DC:0–3 with this revision, the group was authorized to make changes when there was strong evidence in favor of doing so. These changes include the following:

- DC:0–3R no longer includes Gender Identity Disorder because we found no evidence for its meaningful classification in the early years.

- We removed "reactive attachment" from Reactive Attachment Deprivation/Maltreatment Disorder of Infancy. The original label led to confusion on the part of some users of DC:0–3, many of whom believed that the phrase referred to qualitative features of attachment relationships, which would be recorded more appropriately in Axis II. The description of the renamed Deprivation/Maltreatment Disorder includes criteria where none had existed before.

- We renamed Traumatic Stress Disorder as Posttraumatic Stress Disorder, to emphasize congruence with the syndrome that is commonly understood and designated in DSM-IV-TR, and added criteria where none had existed before.

- Regulatory Disorders have been renamed Regulation Disorders of Sensory Processing in order to draw attention to the difficulties in sensory processing that characterize these disorders.

- We include specific Anxiety Disorder subtypes in Anxiety Disorders of Infancy and Early Childhood.

- The Depression of Infancy and Early Childhood category includes two types of depression: Major Depression and Depression NOS.

- Descriptions of Sleep Behavior Disorders and Eating Behavior Disorders incorporate subtypes and criteria from RDC-PA that seem appropriate for toddlers. DC:0–3R notes that Sleep Behavior Disorders can be appropriately classified after 12 months of age, when sleep patterns typically emerge.

- In reviewing Disorders of Relating and Communicating, we took account of considerable clinical research that had taken place since the 1994 publication of DC:0–3. Such research has demonstrated that Autistic Spectrum Disorders can be meaningfully identified in children as young as 2 years of age, thus making the DSM-IV-TR classifications of Pervasive Developmental Disorder, Not Otherwise Specified (PDD-NOS) or Autism more applicable to very young children. DC:0–3R recommends that the use of Multisystem Developmental Disorder (a category that does not require the range of relationship and communication difficulties observed in children with Autistic Disorder) be restricted to children less than 2 years of age.

Most users of Axis II in DC:0–3 relied on the Parent–Infant Relationship Global Assessment Scale (PIR-GAS) to evaluate the quality of a caregiver–child relationship and reach a diagnostic classification, if applicable. DC:0–3R gives the PIR-GAS more prominence by moving it from an appendix to the main text. We also expanded the range of the scale and clarified criteria. We eliminated the Axis II subtypes that appeared in DC:0–3 but included many of their descriptive features in a new Relationship Problems Checklist. The checklist format allows the clinician an opportunity to indicate the extent to which a parent–infant relationship can be described with any of the criterion-based qualities of overinvolved, underinvolved, anxious/tense or angry/hostile.

As in DC:0–3, Axis III of DC:0–3R provides a place to record Medical and Developmental Disorders and other conditions that can be classified using other systems.

Axis IV: Psychosocial Stressors now includes a psychosocial and environmental checklist—similar to what has been found useful in ICD-10—with items appropriate for infants and young children.

Axis V, renamed Emotional and Social Functioning, maintains the perspective of Axis V in DC:0–3, with simplifications designed to enhance its use. We have tried to clarify descriptions of the six capacities for emotional and social functioning identified in DC:0–3 and have given more prominence to the process of rating these capacities.

In DC:0–3, the Introduction included guidelines for selecting an appropriate diagnosis. A revision of this material, entitled "Diagnostic Thinking and Guidelines for Selecting Classifications" appears as Appendix A in DC:0–3R. Many users interpreted the DC: 0–3 guidelines as discouraging the designation of co-occurring diagnostic classifications (or "co-morbidity"). Expert consensus now agrees that the designation of co-occurring diagnostic classifications is appropriate if criteria for each diagnostic classification are met. Appendix A continues to provide guidelines for (1) prioritizing diagnostic classifications on Axis I and (2) identifying a primary diagnosis for purposes of intervention planning. For example, the guidelines stress the importance of prioritizing a diagnosis of Posttraumatic Stress Disorder because of the urgency of providing prompt, comprehensive intervention.

The Future of DC:0–3R

DC:0–3R is designed for use in a new period of clinical application and research concerning the classification of mental health disorders in the earliest years of life. Criteria for classification in DC:0–3R represent the best current thinking of the Revision Task Force and early childhood mental health researchers and clinicians worldwide. We expect that at some future time accumulated experience with DC:0–3R will warrant consideration of a major revision of the system. In anticipation of such a revision, we indicate areas of uncertainty that we can already identify in DC:0–3R, as well as issues that seem important for further study.

Areas of Uncertainty

Revising the original version of a diagnostic classification system within a relatively brief time period requires making judgments about evidence, the integration of differing perspectives, and the usefulness of proposed conceptualizations for clinical trials and application. We hope that many of the decisions we have made have improved the usefulness and developmental appropriateness of the original DC:0–3. Still, we recognize that some of our decisions may not prove useful or appropriate. As noted in the original DC:0–3, as we move forward with a diagnostic classification system, there is an inevitable tension between including descriptions of syndromes based on preliminary clinical consensus and not including them, but rather waiting for systematic research.

Criteria for Subtypes

A related tension exists between specifying criteria for subtypes of a disorder and refraining from doing so. In the absence of clear evidence, should one specify descriptive criteria for subtypes in order to promote research and foster evolution of the system? Given the developmental emphasis of DC:0–3R, we were alert to the hazards of seeking analogues for the problems found in older children in less differentiated infants and toddlers. In other words, when DSM describes subtypes of a disorder seen in children of preschool age or older, should DC:0–3R attempt to identify what subtypes might look like in the early years? Or should the system instead recommend the use of a broader, less-differentiated disorder classification without subtypes?

The Research Task Force went through a decision-making process involving the above dilemmas in considering Anxiety Disorders of Infancy and

Early Childhood. DC:0–3 did not include subtypes. However, we decided to make use of subtypes in DC:0–3R. We were aware of modest evidence suggesting that subtypes of anxiety disorder could be identified in children younger than 4 years of age. Moreover both RDC-PA and DSM-IV-TR specify subtypes of anxiety disorder. Similarly, DC:0–3R includes two subtypes of Depressive Disorders of Infancy and Early Childhood, adopted from RDC-PA. These are Depressive Disorder NOS (Not Otherwise Specified) and Major Depressive Disorder. This subtyping for children less than 4 years old awaits research confirmation. DC:0–3R retains DC:0–3's classification category of Mixed Disorder of Emotional Expressiveness in spite of uncertainty and controversy among clinicians and researchers, some of whom argued that the category could not be sufficiently specified with objective, distinguishable criteria. Other clinicians suggested that retaining the category offered the opportunity for meaningful description by users. DC:0–3R retains the category of Mixed Disorder of Emotional Expressiveness as the field awaits further evidence about its reliability and validity.

Within the category of Regulation Disorders of Sensory Processing ("Regulatory Disorders" in DC:0–3), the Revision Task Force endeavored to clarify subtypes in ways that made conceptual sense according to current clinical thinking. We made use of extensive feedback from our surveys of DC:0–3 users and took advice from a specially convened group of occupational therapists and from other clinicians who had extensive experience using the DC:0–3 classification of Regulatory Disorders. Experts disagreed about the persuasiveness of evidence offered in support of various subtypes and about subtypes' clinical usefulness. As with other subtypes and classifications in DC:0–3R, only future research from clinical trials can identify the classification categories that will prove useful over the long run. The Revision Task Force concluded that at this stage of our knowledge, DC:0–3R could neither provide detailed criteria for subtypes of Regulation Disorders of Sensory Processing nor specify the number of criteria needed for diagnosis. Instead we provided criteria in rich descriptive form in the hope that future research will clarify this area.

DC:0–3R provides criteria for Posttraumatic Stress Disorder that rely on recent empirical evidence and expert consensus. The description of this classification also includes a discussion of "Associated Features" that are not among the criteria required to make a diagnosis of Posttraumatic Stress Disorder. This placement of material reflects the fact that some, but not all, clinicians who work with children younger than 3 years count among the prominent features of Posttraumatic Stress Disorder a temporary loss of previously acquired developmental skills and the appearance of aggression and fears that were not present before the traumatic event.

The classification of Multisystem Developmental Disorder (MSDD) represents another area of uncertainty. Many users of DC:0–3, as well as experts in the identification and investigation of autistic spectrum disorders, told the Revision Task Force this diagnostic classification was unnecessary. They pointed to a lack of evidence to support MSDD as a separate classification. At the same time, a substantial number of DC:0–3 users commented on the usefulness of MSDD and argued for its continued inclusion. As a compromise, DC:0–3R includes MSDD as a diagnostic classification appropriate for children less than 2 years of age. For children 2 years old and older, substantial evidence supports Pervasive Developmental Disorders as a useful framework for identifying and treating autistic spectrum disorders.

Assessing Functional Adaptation

Any evaluation based on the DC:0–3R framework should consider the infant or young child's capacity to participate in meaningful everyday family routines. DC:0–3R addresses the issue of the infant or young child's functional adaptation to the world (independent of diagnosis). In Axis I, depending on the available evidence, some disorders require impairment to meet diagnostic criteria; others do not. Axis II addresses functional adaptation in the context of caregiving relationships. Axis V addresses the quality of functional adaptation in social–emotional development. As is the case with other diagnostic classification systems, functional adaptation criteria are in need of further specification supported by research.

Areas for Further Study

DSM-IV-TR includes an appendix called "Criteria sets and axes provided for further study." In a similar vein, we identify and recommend for study two classifications and an additional axis that are not ready for inclusion in DC:0–3R but that, with additional evidence, might warrant inclusion in a major revision to the DC:0–3 system.

Disruptive Behavior Disorders

A constant challenge in evaluating infants and toddlers is distinguishing developmentally appropriate, relatively normative, and transient levels of disruptive behaviors from early-emerging symptoms of what will become the more differentiated patterns of disruptive behavior disorders of later childhood. Like DC:0–3, DC:0–3R is designed to be sensitive to development in the earliest years of life. Overactivity, poor regulation of impulses, noncompliance, and aggression are common complaints of parents of young children. They are among the most common reasons for clinical referral. These features will often be associated with one of the diagnostic classifications in DC:0–3R. Moreover, it is important to recognize that the ages of 1 to 4 years are a period of rapid developmental change in a child's capacities to regulate emotions and behaviors. The phrase "the terrible twos" reflects popular recognition that young children often have difficulty managing their anger and frustration and may respond to limits or disappointment with defiance or aggressive outbursts. However, these "challenging behaviors" are also among the most common reasons for clinical referral from primary health care providers, child care personnel, and community settings. With the gradual emergence of emotional and social competence, many children's irritability, oppositionality, and aggression decrease, but for other children they are pervasive, persistent, and impairing. For these children, DC:0–3R recommends using the criteria of DSM-IV-TR, as modified by RDC-PA, for Attention-Deficit Hyperactivity Disorder, Conduct Disorder, and Oppositional Defiant Disorder when assessing children of preschool age. There is evidence from a number of studies that syndromes in this group of disorders may appear in children less than 3 years of age.

Excessive Crying Disorder

At the suggestion of some experts in the field, the Revision Task Force considered adding Excessive Crying Disorder as a functional regulatory disorder, along with Sleeping Behavior and Feeding Behavior Disorders. However, neither evidence for criteria nor clinical consensus seemed sufficient to include it in DC:0–3R. It will take longitudinal, developmentally informed study to understand the conditions under which the early, undifferentiated forms of distress seen in infancy and toddlerhood develop—or do not develop—into the more differentiated disorders of childhood.

A Family Axis

We propose the development, circulation for comment, and pilot testing of a Family Axis (Axis VI). This axis would encourage information gathering and appropriate documentation in three areas: (1) family history of mental illness, (2) family structure and available supports, and (3) family culture. Knowledge of these aspects of family life is central to clinical assessment and treatment planning.

Consensus concerning the usefulness of such an axis for clinical formulation is already emerging among clinicians who work with infants, young children, and their families. However, the Revision Task Force did not include an Axis VI in DC:0–3R or even solicit reactions to the idea in surveys of DC:0–3 users. A Family Axis has not been a part of earlier diagnostic classification systems, and we deemed its inclusion in DC:0–3R to exceed the bounds of a minor revision. Still, we hope that future clinical trials will make use of such an axis.

Axis I
Clinical Disorders

---

100. Posttraumatic Stress Disorder

Posttraumatic Stress Disorder describes a pattern of symptoms that may be shown by children who have experienced a single traumatic event, a series of connected traumatic events, or chronic, enduring stress situations. An infant or toddler may directly experience or witness an event or events that involve actual or threatened death or serious injury to the child or others or a threat to the psychological or physical integrity of the child or others.

The trauma may be a sudden and unexpected event (e.g., automobile accident, earthquake, terrorist attack, shooting, mauling by an animal), a series of connected events (e.g., repeated air raids), or an enduring situation (e.g., chronic child battering or sexual abuse). Especially when severe trauma, such as life-threatening injury to the child or to a family member, has occurred, it is important to make the diagnosis and begin working with the child and family immediately if the child's symptoms interfere with aspects of daily functioning and have persisted for at least 1 month.

A child's symptoms must be understood in the context of the trauma, the child's own temperament or personality characteristics, and a caregiver's ability to help the child cope and provide a sense of protection and safety. To understand a child's symptoms, a clinician must appreciate the child's developmental level. In some cases, the memories that children reenact or report may change as part of their attempts to rework the trauma.

The diagnosis of Posttraumatic Stress Disorder requires that **ALL FIVE** of the following criteria be met:

1. The child has been exposed to a traumatic event—that is, an event involving actual or threatened death or serious injury or threat to the physical or psychological integrity of the child or another person.

2. The child shows evidence of reexperiencing the traumatic event(s) by AT LEAST ONE of the following symptoms:

(a) Posttraumatic play—that is, play that (1) represents a reenactment of some aspect of the trauma, (2) is compulsively driven, (3) fails to relieve anxiety, and (4) is more literal and less elaborate and imaginative than usual.

Example: A toddler who was bitten by a dog plays out a scene in which she growls and snarls, then makes sudden lunges. She does not comment on this play and repeats the scene with little variation. An example of *adaptive* play reenactment, in contrast, might be the play of a toddler who was bitten by a dog and then plays out numerous scenes of scary dogs, with different circumstances and outcomes apparent as the content of the play changes over time.

(b) Recurrent and intrusive recollections of the traumatic event outside play—that is, repeated statements or questions about the event that suggest a fascination with the event or preoccupation with some aspect of the event. Distress is not necessarily apparent.

Example: A toddler who was bitten by a dog talks endlessly about dogs and seems drawn to their images in books or on television.

(c) Repeated nightmares, the content of which may or may not be linked to the traumatic event.

(d) Physiological distress, expressed in language or behavior, at exposure to reminders of the trauma.

Example: A parent or caregiver may report feeling that the child's heart is pounding, observe that the child is shaking and trembling, or feel that the child's hands and/or face are sweaty. A young child with verbal skills may report these same physiologic symptoms himself, as well as additional somatic symptoms such as upset stomach, chest tightness, or shortness of breath.

(e) Recurrent episodes of flashbacks or dissociation—that is, reenactment of the event without any sense on the child's part as to the source of the ideas. The behavior is dissociated from the child's intentionality or sense of purpose. This symptom may also present as staring or freezing.

Example: A toddler who is engaged in doll play does not comment on the sound of a siren in the street but abruptly begins a fighting sequence with the dolls, having been reminded of the ambulance which arrived after an argument between her parents.

3. The child experiences a numbing of responsiveness or interference with developmental momentum. The numbing or developmental problem appears or intensifies after the trauma and is revealed by AT LEAST ONE of the following symptoms:

    (a) Increased social withdrawal.

    (b) Restricted range of affect.

    (c) Markedly diminished interest or participation in significant activities, including play, social interactions, and daily routines.

    (d) Efforts to avoid activities, places, or people that arouse recollection of the trauma, including efforts to avoid thoughts, feelings, and conversations associated with the trauma.

  4. After a traumatic event, a child may exhibit symptoms of increased arousal, as revealed by AT LEAST TWO of the following:

    (a) Difficulty going to sleep, evidenced by strong bedtime protest, difficulty falling asleep, or repeated night waking unrelated to nightmares.

    (b) Difficulty concentrating.

    (c) Hypervigilance.

    (d) Exaggerated startle response.

    (e) Increased irritability, outbursts of anger or extreme fussiness, or temper tantrums.

  5. This pattern of symptoms persists for AT LEAST 1 MONTH.

Associated features: Young children who have experienced a traumatic event may temporarily lose previously acquired developmental skills. Aggression toward peers, adults, or animals may appear. Fears not present before the traumatic event may become evident, including separation anxiety, fear of toileting alone, and fear of the dark, among others. Sexual and aggressive behaviors that are inappropriate for the child's age may also be seen.

Note: If a child has been exposed to a traumatic event and the symptoms listed above are present after this event but were not present before it, the diagnosis of Posttraumatic Stress Disorder may be considered primary for purposes of clinical formulation as explained in Appendix A: Diagnostic Thinking and Guidelines for Selecting Classifications.

150. Deprivation/Maltreatment Disorder

This disorder occurs in the context of deprivation or maltreatment, including persistent and severe parental neglect or documented physical or psychological abuse. The disorder may develop when a child has limited opportunity to form selective attachments because of frequent changes of primary caregiver(s) or the marked unavailability of an attachment figure, as in institutional settings. It may also occur when infants and young children are seriously neglected (e.g., by parents who are severely depressed or involved in substance abuse). It is important to note that not all children who are neglected or abused will exhibit this disorder; most will not. Moreover, children may demonstrate symptoms of Deprivation/Maltreatment Disorder when they are not currently deprived of an available caregiver. As part of evaluating the current caregiving environment of a child who has experienced deprivation or maltreatment, the clinician should characterize current caregiving relationships under Axis II and record psychosocial and environmental stressors under Axis IV.

Deprivation/Maltreatment Disorder is characterized by markedly disturbed and developmentally inappropriate attachment behaviors in which a child rarely or minimally turns preferentially to a discriminated attachment figure for comfort, support, protection, and nurturance. Researchers have identified three patterns of Deprivation/Maltreatment Disorder and one rule-out condition.

1. In the **emotionally withdrawn or inhibited pattern**, the child minimally directs attachment behaviors toward adult caregivers. The classification of this pattern requires evidence of THREE OF THE FOLLOWING BEHAVIORS:

   (a) Rarely or minimally seeking comfort in distress.

   (b) Responding minimally to comfort offered to alleviate distress.

   (c) Limited positive affect and excessive levels of irritability, sadness, or fear.

   (d) Reduced or absent social and emotional reciprocity (e.g., reduced affect sharing, social referencing, turn-taking, and eye contact).

2. In the **indiscriminate or disinhibited pattern,** the child directs attachment behaviors nonselectively. The classification of this pattern requires evidence of TWO OF THE FOLLOWING BEHAVIORS:

   (a) Overly familiar behavior and reduced or absent reticence around unfamiliar adults.

   (b) Failure, even in unfamiliar settings, to check back with adult caregivers after venturing away.

   (c) Willingness to go off with an unfamiliar adult with minimal or no hesitation.

3. The diagnosis of Mixed Deprivation/Maltreatment Disorder requires two or more criteria from BOTH 1 AND 2 above.

4. Before making a diagnosis of Deprivation/Maltreatment Disorder, the clinician should be sure that symptoms are not better explained by a Pervasive Developmental Disorder (PDD), a rule-out condition.

Associated Features: Under unusual circumstances, Deprivation/Maltreatment Disorder may be associated with failure to thrive or other growth disturbances, which should be coded separately under Axis III. The diagnostic profile of a child with Deprivation/Maltreatment Disorder will be enriched by information coded under Axis II: Relationship Classification.

200. Disorders of Affect

Disorders of affect reflect an infant's or young child's difficulty with regulation of affects, including depressed mood, anxiety/fear, and anger. Recent evidence from clinical and community studies suggests that disorders of affect are more widespread among infants and young children than had been appreciated. When considering disorders of affect, the clinician must determine whether symptoms are GENERALIZED across settings and relationships or specific to a particular situation or relationship.

210. Prolonged Bereavement/Grief Reaction

The loss of a primary caregiver, particularly a parent, is almost always a serious stressor for an infant or young child. Most young children do not have the emotional and cognitive resources to deal with such a major loss. Moreover, if the grieving child's other caregiver(s) are also grieving, they may not have sufficient emotional resources to respond adequately to the child's need for support.

Manifestations of Prolonged Bereavement/Grief Reaction can include any stage of the sequence of protest, despair, and detachment.

The diagnosis of Prolonged Bereavement/Grief Reaction requires that ALL THREE of the following criteria be met:

1. A child exhibits AT LEAST THREE of the following eight symptoms:
   (a) The child cries, calls, and searches for the absent caregiver.
   (b) The child refuses others' attempts to provide comfort.
   (c) The child withdraws emotionally, evidenced by lethargy, a sad facial expression, and lack of interest in age-appropriate activities.
   (d) Eating is disrupted.
   (e) Sleep is disrupted.
   (f) The child may exhibit arrested development, regression, or loss of previously achieved developmental milestones.
   (g) The child shows diminished range of affect.
   (h) In the face of reminders of the loss, the child shows marked disturbance, for example:
   - Detachment, including seeming indifference toward reminders of the caregiver, such as a photograph or mention of his or her name.

- Selective "forgetting," including apparent lack of recognition of reminders of the caregiver.

- Extreme sensitivity to any reminder of the caregiver, including acute distress when a possession that belonged to the caregiver is touched by another or taken away.

- A strong emotional reaction to any theme remotely connected with separation and loss—for example, refusal to play hide-and-seek or bursting into tears when a household object is moved from its customary place.

2. A change in the child's functioning occurs subsequent to the loss.

3. Symptoms must be present for most of the day, more days than not, over a period of AT LEAST **2 WEEKS**.

220. Anxiety Disorders of Infancy and Early Childhood

A number of the following challenges are involved in efforts to identify anxiety disorders in infants and young children:

- Defining the difference between developmentally expected anxiety or fear and developmentally inappropriate and excessive anxiety, which may be associated with an anxiety disorder. For example, between 7 and 12 months of age, most infants develop a fear of strangers and express distress when separated from their primary caregiver. These fears peak between 9 and 18 months of age and decrease for most children by age 2½.

- Identifying the difference between anxious temperament characteristics and anxiety disorder. A substantial minority of young children can be characterized as "behaviorally inhibited," responding to new people, situations, and objects with fear and withdrawal. Although behaviorally inhibited children may be at increased risk for development of anxiety disorders later in childhood, most will not develop an anxiety disorder.

- Difficulties in assessing young children's anxiety, as infants and toddlers are limited in their verbal and cognitive capacities. Even 3-year-olds may not share their worries and fears with parents and other adults.

Despite these challenges, recent advances in the nosology and diagnosis of psychiatric symptoms and disorders in preschool children have made it possible to begin to define the boundaries among normative anxiety, temperamental variation, and clinically significant anxiety disorders in very young children. Presented below are general characteristics required for the diagnosis of any of the anxiety disorders and diagnostic criteria for specific anxiety disorders in young children. The criteria are adaptations of criteria set forth in the *Diagnostic & Statistical Manual of Mental Disorders* (DSM-IV-TR; American Psychiatric Association, 2000) and RDC-PA (2003) and will be applicable for children ages 2 and older. If a clinician finds strong evidence of impairing anxiety in a child younger than 2, use of the classification Anxiety Disorder Not Otherwise Specified (NOS) is recommended.

General Characteristics of all Anxiety Disorders: The anxiety or fear described in each specific anxiety disorder must meet ALL OF THE FOLLOWING CRITERIA to be considered a possible symptom of an anxiety disorder. The anxiety or fear

- Causes the child distress or leads the child to avoid activities or settings associated with the anxiety or fear.

- Occurs during two or more everyday activities or within two or more relationships (pervasive).

- Is uncontrollable, at least some of the time.

- Impairs the child's or the family's functioning and/or the child's expected development.

- Persists. (*Note:* The criteria for each anxiety disorder specify the minimum duration required for the relevant anxiety to be considered as a symptom of that disorder.)

Associated Feature: Not all young children with an anxiety disorder have a family history of anxiety disorder(s) or depression. However, the presence of a family history of an anxiety or mood disorder is an important associated feature for the majority of young children who meet criteria for an anxiety disorder.

Specific Anxiety Disorders: Listed below are criteria for specific anxiety disorders that can be diagnosed reliably in children 2 years and older. As is the case with older children, particular designated anxiety disorders in young children frequently co-occur with other designated anxiety disorders, as well as with other psychiatric disorders. Co-occurring disorders result in significant psychosocial and developmental impairment.

221. *Separation Anxiety Disorder*

The diagnosis of Separation Anxiety Disorder requires that ALL FIVE of the following criteria be met. Because it is difficult to assess separation anxiety as a disorder in very young children, descriptions of this classification include examples of the presentation of particular symptoms.

1. The child experiences developmentally inappropriate and excessive anxiety concerning separation from home or from those to whom the child is attached. At least some of the time, the child cannot control the anxiety. The anxiety is evidenced by **THREE (OR MORE)** of the following:

   (a) Recurrent, excessive distress when separation from home or major attachment figures occurs or is anticipated.

   Example: Infants, toddlers, and young children may cry persistently and inconsolably and refuse to be cared for and soothed by a substitute caregiver when the parent leaves. They may also engage in aggressive or self-injurious behavior during separation from an attachment figure (e.g., hitting the substitute caregiver or head banging). Persistent, excessive worry about losing major attachment figures or about harm befalling them.

   (b) Persistent, excessive worry that an untoward event (e.g., getting lost or being kidnapped) will lead to separation from a major attachment figure.

   (c) Persistent reluctance or refusal to go to child care, school, or elsewhere out of fear of separation. (*Note:* In very young children, this may appear as (a) fear or anxiety related to leaving home for child care or school, (b) anticipatory fear or anxiety related to child care or school, or (c) resisting or refusing to go to child care or school because of fear or anxiety.)

   (d) Persistent or excessive fear or reluctance to be alone or without major attachment figures at home or without significant adults in other settings.

   Example: A young child may refuse to be alone in a room in her own house and may follow the parent around the house.

   (e) Persistent reluctance or refusal to go to sleep without the presence of a major attachment figure.

   (f) Repeated nightmares involving the theme of separation.

   Note: Preverbal or barely verbal children may have frightening dreams without recognizable content.

   (g) Repeated complaints or expression of physical symptoms when separation from major attachment figures occurs or is anticipated.

   Example: Verbal children may complain about headaches, stomachaches, or nausea. Infants, toddlers, and young children who are anxious about separation from major attachment figures may vomit, hiccup excessively, or drool.

2. The disturbance causes clinically significant distress for the child or leads to avoidance of activities or settings associated with the anxiety or fear.

3. The disturbance impairs the child's or family's functioning and/or the child's expected development.

4. The disturbance does not occur exclusively during the course of pervasive developmental disorder.

5. The disturbance lasts for at least 1 MONTH.

222. *Specific Phobia*

The diagnosis of Specific Phobia requires that ALL SIX of the following criteria be met:

1. The presence or anticipation of a specific object or situation evokes excessive, unreasonable, marked, and persistent fear in the child.

2. Exposure to the phobic stimulus almost invariably provokes an immediate anxiety response in the child, such as panic, crying, tantrums, freezing, or clinging.

3. The child avoids the phobic situation(s) or object or exhibits intense anxiety or distress when contact is unavoidable. Parents may facilitate the young child's avoidance of the phobic situation or object.

4. The child's avoidance, anxious anticipation, or distress in the feared situation(s) causes clinically significant distress or leads to avoidance of activities or settings the child associates with the anxiety or fear. The disturbance impairs the child's or family's functioning and/or the child's expected development.

5. The anxiety or phobic avoidance is not better accounted for by the DSM-IV TR diagnostic category of Obsessive-Compulsive Disorder (e.g., fear of dirt) or by Posttraumatic Stress Disorder (e.g., avoidance of stimuli associated with trauma), Separation Anxiety Disorder (e.g. avoidance of school/daycare), or Social Phobia (e.g., avoidance of social interactions).

6. The disturbance lasts for AT LEAST 4 MONTHS.

223. *Social Anxiety Disorder (Social Phobia)*

The diagnosis of Social Anxiety Disorder requires that ALL SIX of the following criteria be met:

1. The child exhibits marked and persistent fear of one or more social or performance situations that involve exposure to unfamiliar people or possible scrutiny by others. The child must show this fear with both peers and adults. Social or performance situations that evoke fear in young children include play dates with peers, large family gatherings, birthday parties, religious ceremonies, or "circle time" at child care or preschool.

2. Exposure to the feared social situation almost invariably provokes anxiety in the child, who may express anxiety by panic, crying, tantrums, freezing, clinging, or shrinking from social situations with unfamiliar people.

3. The child avoids the feared social or performance situation(s) or endures it with intense anxiety or distress. Parents often protect very young children from the feared situation.

4. The child's avoidance, anxious anticipation, or distress in the feared situation(s) interferes significantly with the child's functioning and/or the child's expected development.

5. The fear or avoidance is not better accounted for by other disorders, including Pervasive Developmental Disorder, Separation Anxiety Disorder, Simple Phobia, or other anxiety disorders.

6. The disturbance lasts for AT LEAST 4 MONTHS.

224. *Generalized Anxiety Disorder*

The diagnosis of Generalized Anxiety Disorder requires that ALL SEVEN of the following criteria be met:

1. The child experiences excessive anxiety and worry more days than not for AT LEAST 6 MONTHS.

2. The child finds it very difficult to control the anxiety or worry (e.g., the child may repeatedly ask a parent for reassurance).

3. The anxiety and/or worry occurs during TWO OR MORE activities or settings or within TWO OR MORE relationships.

4. The anxiety and worry are associated with ONE (OR MORE) of the following six symptoms:

    (a) Restlessness or feeling "keyed up" or "on edge."

    (b) Fatigability.

    (c) Difficulty concentrating.

    (d) Irritability or tantrumming.

    (e) Muscle tension.

    (f) Sleep disturbance (difficulty falling or staying asleep or restless, unsatisfying sleep).

5. The focus of the anxiety or worry is not better accounted for by the DSM-IV-TR diagnostic category of Obsessive-Compulsive Disorder (e.g., fear of dirt or needing ritualized reassurance from a parent), Posttraumatic Stress Disorder, Separation Anxiety Disorder (e.g., anxiety about separation from a caregiver), or Social Phobia (e.g., worry about social interactions).

6. The anxiety, worry, or physical symptoms interfere significantly with the child's functioning and/or the child's expected development.

7. The disturbance is not due to the direct physiologic effect of a substance (e.g., asthma medication or steroids) and does not occur exclusively during a Pervasive Developmental Disorder.

225. Anxiety Disorder Not Otherwise Specified (NOS)

This category includes symptoms of prominent anxiety or phobic avoidance that cause severe distress and/or interfere significantly with functional psychosocial or developmental adaptation. Symptoms do not fully meet the criteria for any *specific* anxiety disorder, but the anxiety or fear of concern must meet ALL FIVE general characteristics for anxiety disorders described in the beginning of this section.

In infants, agitation and/or irritability, uncontrollable crying or screaming, sleeping and eating disturbances, and uncontrollable and pervasive separation distress or social anxiety (particularly in the context of a family history of anxiety disorders or depression) may indicate an early onset anxiety disorder and may be classified as Anxiety Disorder NOS.

When diagnosing Anxiety Disorder, the clinician should keep the following guidelines in mind:

- When trauma is evident or has been reported, and the onset of the child's difficulties follows the trauma, the diagnosis of Posttraumatic Stress Disorder should be considered.

- If the child's anxiety or fear is limited to a particular relationship, a Relationship Classification disorder should be considered.

230. Depression of Infancy and Early Childhood

The criteria for depressive disorders listed below reflect a developmentally sensitive modification of the DSM-IV-TR criteria. As is the case with anxiety disorders, defining and identifying depression in young children presents significant challenges, particularly because young children may not have the verbal or cognitive skills to describe their feelings or emotional experiences.

To diagnose a depressive disorder in a very young child, the clinician must observe ALL FIVE of these general characteristics:

1. The disturbed affect and pattern of behavior should represent a change from the child's baseline mood and behavior.

2. The depressed/irritable mood or anhedonia must be persistent and, at least some of the time, uncoupled from sad or upsetting experiences

(e.g., watching a sad television show, being punished). "Persistent" means being PRESENT FOR MOST OF THE DAY, MORE DAYS THAN NOT, OVER A PERIOD OF AT LEAST 2 WEEKS.

3. Symptoms should be pervasive, occurring in more than one activity or setting and in more than one relationship. If depressive symptoms occur only within one relationship, a diagnosis under Axis II: Relationship Classification should be considered.

4. Symptoms should be causing the child clear distress, impairing functioning, or impeding development.

5. Disturbances are not due to a general medical condition (e.g., hypothyroidism) or the direct effect of a substance (e.g., medication, toxin).

231. Type I: Major Depression

A diagnosis of Major Depression requires that FIVE of the following symptoms must be present **most of the day,** *more days than not,* for AT LEAST 2 WEEKS and MUST INCLUDE ONE OF THE FIRST TWO SYMPTOMS:

1. Depressed or irritable mood most of the day, more days than not, as indicated by either the child's direct expression (e.g., "I'm sad") or observations made by others (e.g., the child appears sad or is tearful).

2. Markedly diminished pleasure or interest in all, or almost all, activities, such as initiation of play and interaction with caregivers, more days than not (as indicated either by child report or observations made by others; e.g. "Nothing (or almost nothing) is fun.").

3. Significant weight loss or gain (e.g. a change of more than 5% of body weight in a month, or significant decrease or increase in appetite, or failure to make expected weight gains.

4. Insomnia or hypersomnia.

5. Psychomotor agitation or retardation that is observable by others (not merely a child's subjective feelings of restlessness or being "slowed down").

6. Fatigue or loss of energy.

7. Evidence of feelings of worthlessness or inappropriate guilt in play (e.g., self-punitive actions and play) or in the child's direct expression.

8. Diminished ability to think or concentrate or indecisiveness (either by subjective account or as observed by others) for several days. In younger children, these symptoms may appear as difficulty in solving problems, responding to caregivers, and/or sustaining attention.

9. Recurrent allusions to or themes of death or suicide or attempts at self-harm. The child may demonstrate these symptoms through thoughts, activities, play, or potentially lethal behaviors.

232. Type II: Depressive Disorder NOS

The diagnosis of Type II: Depressive Disorder NOS requires the presence of THREE OR FOUR OF THE NINE SYMPTOMS described for Type I: Major Depression above. Symptoms must be present for A MINIMUM OF 2 WEEKS. The diagnosis requires the presence of AT LEAST ONE of the first two symptoms.

Associated Feature: When symptoms of Major Depression or Depressive Disorder NOS are observed in the presence of significant psychosocial/ environmental deprivation, the clinician should note these circumstances and consider Deprivation/Maltreatment Disorder of Infancy as an alternative classification, especially if the deprivation is severe.

If the clinician observes symptoms of Major Depression or Depressive Disorder NOS in the presence of significant trauma (see Criteria 1 under Posttraumatic Stress Disorder), these circumstances should be noted and Posttraumatic Stress Disorder considered as the primary diagnosis. Similarly, if the clinician observes symptoms of Major Depression or Depressive Disorder NOS in a child who has lost a primary caregiver, Prolonged Bereavement/Grief Reaction should be considered as an alternative diagnosis. If depressive symptoms are not severe and appear in the context of an adjustment that the child is in the process of making (e.g., adjustment to a parent's beginning full-time work outside the home), the clinician should consider a classification of Adjustment Disorder.

240. Mixed Disorder of Emotional Expressiveness

Mixed Disorder of Emotional Expressiveness is characterized by a child's difficulty in expressing a developmentally appropriate range and intensity of emotions over AT LEAST A 2-WEEK PERIOD. The pattern is pervasive, across multiple types of affect, and represents a change from the child's previous functioning. The diagnosis requires the presence of AT LEAST ONE OF THE FIRST TWO SYMPTOMS listed below AND interference with age-appropriate functioning (third symptom below). When a child exhibits developmental delays, the clinician should use this classification only if the disturbance in affective expression is inappropriate to the child's developmental level. Criteria are:

1. The absence or near-absence of TWO OR MORE specific affects (e.g., pleasure, anger, fear, curiosity, sadness, and excitement) that are expectable given the child's age. The child's difficulty in using language or play to express emotions supports this classification. The clinician may observe a notable absence of age-expectable fears, concerns, or anxieties, such as fears of separation or bodily harm, that serve adaptive functioning.

2. Disturbed intensity of affect, reversed affect or affect inappropriate to the situation

   (a) Disturbed intensity of emotional expression, such as outbursts of anger or blandness and apathy.

   (b) Reversal of affect or affect inappropriate to the situation, such as "silliness" or laughing with apparent bravado when negative emotions, such as fear or remorse, would be appropriate.

3. Interference with appropriate functioning.

300. Adjustment Disorder

The diagnosis of Adjustment Disorder should be considered for any transient situational disturbances that (1) do not meet the criteria for other Axis I diagnoses (such as Posttraumatic Stress Disorder or Prolonged Bereavement/Grief Reaction), (2) are not merely an exacerbation of another preexisting disorder, and (3) do not represent developmentally appropriate reactions to changes in the environment.

The diagnosis of Adjustment Disorder requires that ALL FOUR of the following criteria be met:

1. An environmental stressor event or events (such as those listed in Axis IV: Psychosocial Stressors) is present.

2. A disturbance of affect or behavior appears WITHIN 1 MONTH of the environmental stressor event(s). The infant or young child may exhibit affective symptoms (appearing, for example, subdued, irritable, sober, anxious, or withdrawn) or behavioral symptoms (for example, oppositionality, resistance to going to sleep, frequent tantrums, or regression in toilet training) or both.

3. Symptoms do not meet criteria for Posttraumatic Stress Disorder, Disorders of Affect, or Disorders of Relating and Communicating.

4. Symptoms persist for MORE THAN 2 WEEKS.

400. Regulation Disorders of Sensory Processing

Regulation Disorders of Sensory Processing are constitutionally based responses to sensory stimuli. The diagnosis of Regulation Disorders of Sensory Processing refers to a child's difficulties in regulating emotions and behaviors as well as motor abilities in response to sensory stimulation that lead to impairment in development and functioning. The patterns of behavior that are characteristic of this disorder are manifest (1) across settings and (2) within multiple relationships. The infant or young child's patterns of behavior may affect daily functioning, including interactions with adults and other children.

Sensory stimuli include touch, sight, sound, taste, smell, sensation of movement in space, and awareness of the position of one's body in space. Every child has specific ways of responding to sensory stimuli in the environment. Some children have difficulty processing sensory input and regulating their responses. Difficulties in sensory processing and regulating responses may interfere with a child's overall social and emotional development and motor ability and, more specifically, with the child's ability to participate in age-appropriate activities.

Caregivers moderate a child's behavioral responses to sensory input. Caregivers who are attuned to the child's patterns of behavior can ameliorate the child's regulation difficulties. On the other hand, mismatches between a child's constitutional responses to sensory stimuli and caregiver patterns may intensify such regulation difficulties.

The diagnosis of Regulation Disorders of Sensory Processing includes the presence of THREE FEATURES: (1) sensory processing difficulties, (2) motor difficulties, and (3) a specific behavioral pattern.

If all three features are not characteristic of a child, the clinician should consider alternative classifications. For example:

• Negative and "willful" behavior may arise from coercive parenting (Axis II: Relationship Classification).

• Negative and "willful" behavior may reflect a primary disruptive behavior disorder, such as Oppositional Defiant Disorder (DSM-IV-TR, 2000), that is not specifically associated with sensory processing difficulties.

• Fearfulness, as described in Type A: Hypersensitivity Regulation Disorder (described below), may reflect an Anxiety Disorder.

Regulation Disorders of Sensory Processing may co-occur with other disorders (e.g., Type A: Hypersensitive Regulation Disorders of Sensory Processing and Separation Anxiety Disorder). Symptoms of the Regulation Disorder and the co-occurring disorder(s) may overlap to some degree.

Three types of Regulation Disorders of Sensory Processing, one of which includes two subtypes, are described. Each description identifies specific behavioral, sensory, and motor patterns that characterize the type or subtype. Although there is broad consensus concerning the usefulness of these classifications, specific criteria have not been identified at this stage of our knowledge.

410: Hypersensitive

Infants or toddlers who are hypersensitive to sensory stimuli experience them as aversive. Stimuli that frequently trigger aversive behaviors include light touch, loud noises, bright lights, unfamiliar smells and tastes, rough textures, and/or movement in space.

An infant or young child with a regulation disorder arising from hypersensitivity to various stimuli will show one of two characteristic patterns of behavior:

- Type A: Fearful/Cautious or
- Type B: Negative/Defiant.

Children with either pattern of behavior avoid or demonstrate aversive reactions to sensory stimuli. In other words, fearful/cautious infants and young children and negative/defiant infants and young children have the same underlying pattern of hypersensitivity to stimuli, even though their behavioral patterns differ.

Hypersensitive children have difficulty modulating their responses to sensory input. They are easily overwhelmed by the sensory stimuli that are part of everyday life, and they tend to experience considerable stress as they try to manage their intense responses to such stimuli. Behavioral responses to various stimuli may vary, depending on: (1) the intensity, duration, or location of the stimulus (e.g., a child may tolerate a single stimulus but respond aversively to subsequent stimuli of the same type), (2) a child's baseline level of arousal (e.g., a child may be calm and alert in the morning but become overexcited when she is tired at the end of the day), (3) the source of the stimulus (e.g., a child may respond to self-initiated touch differently than imposed touch).

It is also important to note that Type A: Fearful/Cautious Hypersensitivity may co-occur with Anxiety Disorders and that Type B: Negative/Defiant Hypersensitivity may co-occur with disruptive behavior disorders such as Oppositional Defiant Disorder.

411: Type A: Fearful/Cautious

1. Sensory Reactivity Patterns

   (a) These patterns are characterized by overreactivity to sensory stimuli, including light touch, loud noises, bright lights, unfamiliar smells and tastes, rough textures, or movement in space.

   Example: A toddler may not be able to tolerate rough-and-tumble play or swinging. An infant may signal distress when placed in a supine position or shifted in position (particularly if the head is tipped back).

   (b) Responses to sensory stimuli may include:
   - Fearfulness.
   - Crying.
   - "Freezing."

- Attempted escape from the stimulus.
- Increased distractibility.
- Aggression.
- Angry outbursts, including tantrums.
- Excessive startle reactions.
- Motoric agitation.
- Restricted tolerance for variety in food textures, tastes, and smells.

2. Motor Patterns

Hypersensitivity and aversion to sensory stimuli may limit the child's experience in manipulating or interacting with the environment, resulting in functional deficits in motor development. Motor patterns, which vary among children, may include:

(a) Difficulties with postural control and tone.

(b) Difficulty in fine motor coordination (often associated with play and experience with toys and other objects that have been limited by the child's hypersensitivity).

(c) Difficulty with motor planning.

(d) Less exploration than expected for age.

(e) Limited sensory-motor play.

3. Behavioral Patterns

Behavioral patterns of infants and young children with Type A: Fearful/ Cautious Hypersensitivity include excessive cautiousness, inhibition, and fearfulness. In addition to these patterns, the behavior patterns of *infants* with Type A: Hypersensitivity may include:

(a) Restricted range of exploration.

(b) Limited assertiveness.

(c) Distress when routines change.

(d) Fear and clinginess in new situations.

The behavior patterns of *toddlers and preschoolers* with Type A: Hypersensitivity may also include:

(a) Excessive fears or worries or both.

(b) Shyness in response to new people, places, or objects in the environment.

(c) Distractibility by sensory stimuli.

(d) Impulsivity when overloaded by sensory stimuli.

(e) Frequent periods of irritability and tearfulness.

(f) Limited ability to self-soothe (e.g., difficulty returning to sleep after waking).

- Difficulty recovering from frustration or disappointment.
- Avoidance or slow engagement in new experiences or sensations.

412: *Type B: Negative/Defiant*

1. Sensory reactivity patterns are identical to those of Type A.
2. Motor patterns are also identical to those described in Type A: Fearful/Cautious.
3. Behavioral patterns in Type B, however, are different from those in Type A.

The child with Negative/Defiant Hypersensitivity tends to avoid or be slow to engage in new experiences and, in general, is aggressive only when provoked. The behavior patterns of infants and young children with Type B: Negative/Defiant Hypersensitivity include:

(a) Negativistic behavior (e.g., in an infant, persistent fussiness; in a toddler or preschooler, reflexive negative responses to parental requests or frequent angry outbursts, including tantrums).
(b) Controlling behaviors.
(c) Defiance (behavior the opposite of what is requested or expected).
(d) Preference for repetition, absence of change, and, if change is necessary, change at a slow pace.
(e) Difficulty adapting to changes in routines or plans.
(f) Compulsiveness and perfectionism.
(g) Avoidance or slow engagement in new experiences or sensations.

420: Hyposensitive/Underresponsive

Infants, toddlers, and young children who are hyposensitive require high-intensity sensory input before they are able to respond. Children who are hyposensitive are generally quiet and watchful. They often seem unresponsive to their environment and unreceptive to overtures from others. Significant effort or persistence or both may be needed to engage a hyposensitive child. Although children who are hyposensitive may appear sad or uninterested in their surroundings, their withdrawal and lack of responsivity usually reflect their failure to reach the threshold of arousal that would motivate them to act and interact.

In considering a diagnosis of Hyposensitive/Underresponsive Regulation Disorder, the clinician must be careful to determine that (1) the child's limited social responsivity does not reflect the impairment of social engagement characteristic of Pervasive Developmental Disorders, (2) the child's withdrawal does not reflect depressed mood, as in Major Depression or a Depressive Disorder, and (3) the child's withdrawal is not a symptom of an anxiety disorder, such as Social Anxiety Disorder.

1. Sensory Reactivity Patterns
   (a) Underreactivity to sounds, movement, smell, taste, touch, and proprioception.
   (b) In infants, lack of responsivity to sensations and social overtures.

2. Motor Patterns
   (a) Limited exploration.
   (b) Restricted play repertoire.
   (c) Search for specific sensory input, often found in repetitive sensory activities, such as swinging or jumping up and down on a bed.
   (d) Lethargy.
   (e) Poor motor planning and clumsiness, caused by a poorly developed body schema—a consequence of underreactivity to tactile and proprioceptive input.

3. Behavioral Patterns
   (a) Apparent lack of interest in exploring properties of objects, playing challenging games, or engaging in social interactions.
   (b) Apathetic appearance.
   (c) Fatigability.
   (d) Withdrawal from stimuli.
   (e) Inattentiveness.

In addition to the above symptoms, *infants* with Hyposensitive/ Underresponsive Regulation Disorder may appear delayed or depressed. *Preschoolers* with the disorder may "tune out" from conversation and may reveal only a limited range of ideas and fantasies in everyday behavior or imaginative play.

430: Sensory Stimulation-Seeking/Impulsive

Infants, toddlers, and young children who seek out sensory stimulation, like children who are hyposensitive, require high-intensity, frequent, and/or long-duration sensory input before they are able to respond. Unlike hyperactive children, these infants, toddlers, and preschoolers actively seek to satisfy their need for high levels of sensory input much more of the time than typically developing children. This pattern of sensory and motor reactivity may be associated with Attention-Deficit Hyperactivity Disorder (DSM-IV-TR), particularly the hyperactive/impulsive type or combined type.

1. Sensory Reactivity Patterns
    (a) Craving for high-intensity sensory stimuli. Such a craving may lead to destructive or high-risk behaviors.

2. Motor Patterns
    (a) High need for motor discharge.
    (b) Diffuse impulsivity.
    (c) Accident proneness without clumsiness.

3. Behavioral patterns
    (a) High activity levels.
    (b) Seeking constant contact with people and objects.
    (c) Seeking stimulation through deep pressure.
    (d) Recklessness.
    (e) Disorganized behavior as a consequence of sensory stimulation.

In addition to the symptoms above, infants may also seek or crave sensory input and stimulation.

In addition to the symptoms above, preschoolers may also be

- Excitable.
- Aggressive.
- Intrusive.
- Daring and reckless, risking accidents and injuries.
- Preoccupied with aggressive themes in pretend play.

Not infrequently, the sensory stimulation-seeking child's urgent need for physical contact with people or objects leads to destruction of property, intrusion into others' physical space, or hitting without apparent provocation. Children and adults may mistake the sensory stimulation-seeking child's excitability for aggression. Once others react aggressively to the child, the child may begin to behave aggressively with intention.

500. Sleep Behavior Disorder

Sleep problems are common during the first year of life. They are associated with a variety of conditions and medical problems. The clinician should not use this diagnosis when a young child's sleep problem is primarily due to disorders of affect, transient adjustment problems, Posttraumatic Stress Disorder, or a relationship disorder.

The classification of Sleep Behavior *Disorder* is reserved for two types of conditions that occur after 12 months of age, when stable sleep patterns typically emerge. Following the recommendations of the RDC-PA (2003), we distinguish two forms of Sleep Behavior Disorder for the toddler and young child. These supplement the classifications in DSM-IV-TR (2000) that include: sleep terrors, sleepwalking disorder, breathing-related sleep disorder, and nightmare disorder. If criteria are met for DSM-IV-TR classifications in a young child, the appropriate diagnosis should be coded under Axis I (800, "Other") in DC:0–3R.

The supplemental classifications in DC:0–3R are:

- Sleep-Onset Protodyssomnia—Disorders of initiating sleep.
- Night-Waking Protodyssomnia—Disorders of maintaining sleep (e.g., waking up during the night, with difficulty returning to sleep).

510. Sleep-Onset Disorder (Sleep-Onset Protodyssomnia)

Sleep-onset problems are reflected in the time it takes a child to fall asleep, the child's need for the parent to stay in the room until she falls asleep, and/or the child's need for reunions with the parent (i.e., the parent leaves the room and comes back in response to bids from the child).

The diagnosis of Sleep-Onset Disorder requires that there be significant difficulty falling asleep for AT LEAST 4 WEEKS, with five to seven episodes per week.

The child must be 12 months of age or older.

520. Night-Waking Disorder (Night-Waking Protodyssomnia)

Night-waking problems are reflected in awakenings that require parental intervention and/or removal to the parental bed.

A diagnosis of Night-Waking Disorder requires that significant difficulty in nighttime awakenings be present for AT LEAST 4 WEEKS and involve five to seven episodes per week.

The child must be 12 months of age or older.

600. Feeding Behavior Disorder

The diagnosis of Feeding Behavior Disorder, the symptoms of which may become evident at different stages of infancy and early childhood, should be considered when an infant or young child has difficulty establishing regular feeding patterns—that is, when the child does not regulate his feeding in accordance with physiological feelings of hunger or fullness. If these difficulties occur in the absence of hunger and/or interpersonal precipitants such as separation, negativism, or trauma, the clinician should consider a primary feeding disorder.

Specific feeding disorders of infancy and early childhood such as pica and rumination are described in DSM-IV-TR. As in the RDC-PA, criteria are listed here for six subcategories of Feeding Behavior Disorder.

601. *Feeding Disorder of State Regulation*

The diagnosis of Feeding Disorder of State Regulation requires that ALL THREE of the following criteria be met:

 (1)   The infant has difficulty reaching and maintaining a calm state during feeding(e.g., the infant is too sleepy, too agitated, and/or too distressed to feed).

 (2)   Feeding difficulties start in the newborn period.

 (3)   The infant fails to gain weight or loses weight.

602. *Feeding Disorder of Caregiver–Infant Reciprocity*

The diagnosis of Feeding Disorder of Caregiver–Infant Reciprocity requires that ALL THREE of the following criteria be met:

 (1)   The infant or young child does not display developmentally appropriate signs of social reciprocity (e.g., visual engagement, smiling, or babbling) with the primary caregiver during feeding.

 (2)   The infant or young child shows significant growth deficiency.

 (3)   The growth deficiency and lack of relatedness are not due solely to a physical disorder or a pervasive developmental disorder.

603. *Infantile Anorexia*

The diagnosis of Infantile Anorexia requires that ALL SIX of the following criteria be met:

 (1)   The infant or young child refuses to eat adequate amounts of food for at least 1 month.

 (2)   Onset of the food refusal occurs before the child is 3 years old.

 (3)   The infant or young child does not communicate hunger and lacks interest in food but shows strong interest in exploration, interaction with caregiver, or both.

 (4)   The child shows significant growth deficiency.

 (5)   The food refusal does not follow a traumatic event.

 (6)   The food refusal is not due to an underlying medical illness.

604. Sensory Food Aversions

The diagnosis of Sensory Food Aversions requires that ALL FOUR of the following criteria be met:

  (1) The child consistently refuses to eat specific foods with specific tastes, textures, and/or smells.

  (2) Onset of the food refusal occurs during the introduction of a novel type of food (e.g., the child may drink one type of milk but refuse another, may eat carrots but refuse green beans, may drink milk but refuse baby food).

  (3) The child eats without difficulty when offered preferred foods.

  (4) The food refusal causes specific nutritional deficiencies or delay of oral motor development.

605. Feeding Disorder Associated with Concurrent Medical Condition

The diagnosis of Feeding Disorder Associated with Concurrent Medical Condition requires that ALL FOUR of the following criteria be met:

  (1) The infant or young child readily initiates feeding, but shows distress over the course of feeding and refuses to continue feeding.

  (2) The child has a concurrent medical condition that the CLINICIAN JUDGES to be the cause of the distress.

  (3) Medical management improves but does not fully alleviate the feeding problem.

  (4) The child fails to gain adequate weight or may even lose weight.

606. Feeding Disorder Associated with Insults to the Gastrointestinal Tract

The diagnosis of Feeding Disorder Associated with Insults to the Gastrointestinal Tract requires that ALL FOUR of the following criteria be met:

  (1) Food refusal follows a major aversive event or repeated noxious insults to the oropharynx or gastrointestinal tract (e.g., choking, severe vomiting, reflux, insertion of nasogastric or endotracheal tubes, suctioning) that trigger intense distress in the infant or young child.

  (2) The infant or young child's consistent refusal to eat takes one of the following forms:

    (a) The infant or young child refuses to drink from the bottle but may accept food offered by spoon. (Although the child may consistently refuse to drink from the bottle when awake, she may drink from the bottle when sleepy or asleep.)

(b) The infant or young child refuses solid food but may accept the bottle.

(c) The child refuses all oral feedings.

(3) Reminders of the traumatic event(s) cause distress, as manifested by one or more of the following:

(a) The infant shows anticipatory distress when positioned for feeding.

(b) The infant or young child resists intensely when a caregiver approaches with a bottle or food.

(c) The infant or young child shows intense resistance to swallowing food placed in her mouth.

(4) The food refusal poses an acute or long-term threat to the child's nutrition.

Note: This diagnosis should not be used when a young child's feeding problem is primarily due to Disorders of Affect, Adjustment Disorder, Posttraumatic Stress Disorder, Deprivation/Maltreatment Disorder, or a Relationship Disorder.

If organic/structural problems (e.g., cleft palate, reflux) affect the child's ability to eat or digest food, the clinician should not use Feeding Behavior Disorder as a primary diagnosis. The clinician can indicate the appropriate medical diagnosis under Axis III. However, if a feeding disturbance that originated from organic or structural difficulties continues after these initial difficulties have been resolved, the diagnosis of Feeding Behavior Disorder may be appropriate.

700. Disorders of Relating and Communicating

This group of disorders is first evident in infancy and early childhood. These disorders involve severe difficulties in relating and communicating, combined with difficulties in the regulation of physiological, sensory, attentional, motor, cognitive, somatic, and affective processes.

In DSM-IV-TR, Disorders of Relating and Communicating are referred to as Pervasive Developmental Disorders. They include Autistic Disorder, Childhood Disintegrative Disorder, Asperger's Disorder, Rhett's Disorder, and Pervasive Developmental Disorder Not Otherwise Specified (PDD-NOS). A growing body of clinical evidence suggests that children who are currently being diagnosed with Pervasive Developmental Disorder present a range of relationship patterns, differences in affect regulation, and a variety of processing and cognitive difficulties. Until recently, only children with the most severe types of difficulties in relating and communicating were described as evidencing Autistic Disorder. An expanded diagnostic framework has now emerged, with Autistic Disorder now seen as one of a group of disorders that have characteristics in common but are distinguished from one another by variations in severity of symptoms across various developmental domains. Autistic Disorder can be diagnosed as early as 2 years of age. DC:0–3R includes a classification of Multisystem Developmental Disorder (MSDD) that can be applied to some children under 2 years of age. MSDD is based on a conceptualization that does not require the range of relationship and communication difficulties observed in clinical populations of children with Autistic Disorder. At this stage of our knowledge, the features of MSDD are descriptive rather than criterion-based.

Children whose symptoms meet the DSM-IV-TR criteria for any of the categories of Pervasive Developmental Disorder (PDD), including PDD-NOS, should have the appropriate diagnosis recorded on DC:0–3R as an 800 diagnosis (e.g., 700 [Autistic Disorder 299.00]; 700 [PDD-NOS 299.80]).

710. Multisystem Developmental Disorder (MSDD)

Some clinicians may prefer to use the diagnosis of MSDD rather than PDD-NOS for infants or toddlers less than 2 years old who have the following characteristics:

- Significant impairment in the ability to engage in an emotional and social relationship with a primary caregiver (e.g., the child may appear avoidant or aimless but may evidence subtle, emergent forms of relating or relate quite warmly intermittently).

- Significant impairment in forming, maintaining, and/or developing preverbal gestural communication or verbal and nonverbal symbolic communication.

- Significant dysfunction in the processing of visual, auditory, tactile, proprioceptive, and vestibular sensations, including hyperreactivity and hyporeactivity to sensory input.

- Significant dysfunction in motor planning (sequencing movements).

Infants and toddlers diagnosed with MSDD have four areas of difficulty that may change as development progresses. Descriptors for each area suggest the range of observable behaviors:

1. Relatedness

   (a) Aimless and mostly unconnected.

   (b) Intermittently connected.

   (c) Often connected.

2. Communications

   (a) Few consistent simple intentional gestures.

   (b) Intermittent simple intentional gestures.

   (c) Consistent intermittent intentional gestures.

   (d) Language use (single words to simple sentences).

3. Affect

   (a) Flat or inappropriate.

   (b) Fleeting satisfaction and pleasure.

   (c) Intermittent aloofness.

   (d) Evident pleasure in interactions.

4. Sensory Processing

   (a) Self-stimulation and rhythmic behavior; both under- and over-reactivity.

   (b) Intermittent organization of behavior; mixed pattern of sensory reactivity.

   (c) Frequent organization of behavior; beginnings of integration.

800. Other Disorders (DSM-IV-TR or ICD 10)

This coding is to be used for other mental health–related classifications not found in DC:0–3R that are found in DSM-IV-TR or ICD 10. Medical diagnoses and major developmental disabilities are to be listed under Axis III on DC:0–3R and relationship classifications under Axis II.

Axis II
Relationship Classification

Understanding the quality of the parent–infant relationship is a required part of developing a diagnostic profile for infants, toddlers, and young children. Primary relationships—such as relationships between an infant or young child and a few familiar adults who take responsibility for the child's care and well-being—provide infants and toddlers with the individualized support they need for healthy development. Within the context of caregiving relationships, the infant builds a sense of what is expected and what is possible in relationships with other people. The infant learns skills and discovers incentives for social initiation, reciprocity, and cooperation. In repeated interactions with emotionally available caregivers, the young child begins to develop the capacity for autonomous emotional regulation and self-control.

When a relationship disorder exists, it is ***specific to a relationship***. The relationship classifications of Axis II identify the types of disturbances that clinicians are likely to see in specific relationships and in interactions between infants and young children and their parents. The clinician should consider and conceptualize primary relationships as entities to be assessed and, when indicated, diagnosed. A skilled clinician can use the concepts and measures in Axis II to formulate and focus interventions for the child, the adult, and their relationship.

In assessing the parent-infant relationship, the clinician should consider multiple aspects of the relationship dynamic, including:

1. Overall functional level of both the child and the parent.
2. Level of distress in both the child and the parent.
3. Adaptive flexibility of both the child and the parent.
4. Level of conflict and resolution between the child and the parent.
5. Effect of the quality of the relationship on the child's developmental progress.

The PIR-GAS and the RPCL

Axis II offers the clinician two tools for evaluating a Relationship Classification under Axis II:

1. The *Parent–Infant Relationship Global Assessment Scale (PIR-GAS)* and
2. The *Relationship Problems Checklist (RPCL)*.

The PIR-GAS allows for a judgment about the relationship classification under consideration. On the PIR-GAS scale, the quality of the infant–parent relationship, ranges from well adapted to severely impaired. The clinician typically completes the scale after multiple clinical evaluations for a referred problem. Clinicians who use the PIR-GAS should remember that relationship problems may or may not co-occur with symptomatic behaviors in the infant. In other words, an infant may have symptoms of a serious mental health disorder and yet have adaptive, flexible relationships with parents and other important adults. Diagnoses of relationship disturbances or disorders are made not only on the basis of observed behavior but also on the basis of parent's subjective experience of the child as expressed during a clinical interview and the subjective experience of the child, as expressed in a play interview, for example. When difficulties in the focal relationship are apparent, the clinician assesses the **intensity**, **frequency,** and **duration** of the difficulties in order to classify the relationship problem as a perturbation, a disturbance, or a disorder.

PIR-GAS scores are classified as:

81–100—Adapted Relationship
41–80—Features of a Disordered Relationship
0–40—Disordered Relationship

A PIR-GAS score below 40 indicates a relationship disorder (and hence should be coded as such on Axis II). However, many parent–infant relationships with a PIR-GAS score between 40 and 80 may show tendencies toward, or features of, a disordered relationship that may benefit from therapeutic intervention.

It is not necessary to know the etiology of current relationship problems in order to use the scale. Symptoms may derive from conditions within the infant, from within the caregiver, from the unique "fit" between infant and caregiver, from the larger social context, or from a combination of several of these factors. The clinician who understands the stressors that are affecting a parent–child relationship may know a great deal about the origins of the problem. Moreover, coding of the infant/young child–parent relationship on the PIR-GAS does not imply that the current nature and quality of the parent–child relationship is immutable. PIR-GAS scores are meant to capture the nature of the relationship at time of assessment. Scores may vary over time, as the quality of a relationship is subject to numerous factors, both intrinsic and extrinsic to the relationship, including therapeutic intervention. Additionally, a clinician should be aware of how particular developmental stages in the child may adversely interact with a parent's experiences, expectations, or challenges to produce disturbances in the child–parent relationship. These disturbances may evolve or go into remission as the child (or the parent) changes.

The Relationship Problems Checklist (RPCL) is intended to help the clinician document the problems or lack of problems in a relationship. The RPCL is not designed as a diagnostic tool. Rather, it enables the clinician to record the extent to which "overinvolved," "underinvolved," "anxious/ tense" and "angry/hostile" are useful descriptors of a given caregiver–infant relationship. The RPCL also lists categories of abuse and neglect.

The clinician should use the PIR-GAS and RPCL to assess the relationship between primary caregiver(s) and the infant or young child. Primary caregivers may be biological, foster, and adoptive parent(s), as well as grandparents, members of the extended family, and caregivers outside the family.

The Parent–Infant Relationship Global Assessment Scale (PIR-GAS)

PIR-GAS Ratings

91–100 Well Adapted

Parent–child relationships in this range are functioning exceptionally well. They are mutually enjoyable and without sustained distress. They evidence adaptation to new circumstances and are typically free of conflict as parent and child manage the stresses of everyday life. The relationship clearly promotes the growth of both child and parent.

81–90 Adapted

Relationships in this range are also functioning well, without evidence that the relationship is significantly stressful for either partner. Interactions within these relationships are frequently reciprocal and synchronous, without distress, and reasonably adaptive. At times parent and child may be in substantial conflict, but conflicts do not persist longer than a few days and are resolved with appropriate consideration of the child's developmental status. The pattern of the relationship protects and promotes the developmental progress of both child and parent.

71–80 Perturbed

Some aspect of the overall functioning of relationships in this range is less than optimal; child and parent may experience transient distress lasting up to a few weeks. Nevertheless, the relationship remains characterized by adaptive flexibility. The disturbance is limited to one domain of functioning. Overall, the relationship still functions reasonably well and does not impede developmental progress.

61–70 Significantly Perturbed

Relationships in this range of functioning are strained but still largely adequate and satisfying to the partners. Conflicts are limited to one or two problematic areas. Both parent and child may experience distress and difficulty for a month or more. The relationship maintains adaptive flexibility, as parent and child seem likely to negotiate the challenge to their relationship successfully. A parent may be stressed by the perturbation, but is not generally overconcerned about the changed relationship pattern, considering it within the range of expectable, relatively short-lived difficult periods in a lifelong relationship.

51–60 Distressed

Relationships in this range of functioning are more than transiently affected as one or both partners experience distress in the context of their relationship. Parent and child maintain some flexibility and adaptive qualities, but conflict may spread across multiple domains of functioning, and resolution is difficult. The developmental progress of the dyad seems likely to falter if the pattern does not improve. Caregivers may or may not be concerned about the disturbed relationship pattern. Neither parent nor child is likely to show overt symptoms resulting from the disturbance.

41–50 Disturbed

The adaptive qualities of a disturbed relationship are beginning to be overshadowed by problematic features. Although not deeply entrenched, dysfunctional patterns appear more than transient. Developmental progress can still proceed, but may be temporarily interrupted.

31–40 Disordered

Rigidly maladaptive interactions, particularly if they involve distress in one or both partners, are the hallmark of disordered relationships. Most interactions between partners are conflicted; some relationships without overt conflicts may nevertheless be grossly inappropriate developmentally. Developmental progress of the child and the parent–child relationship is likely to be influenced adversely.

21–30 Severely Disordered

Relationships in this range of functioning are severely compromised. Both parent and child are significantly distressed by the relationship itself. Maladaptive interactive patterns are rigidly entrenched. To an observer, interactive patterns seem to have been in place for a long time, although the onset may have been insidious. In a severely disordered relationship, a significant proportion of interactions are likely to be conflicted. Developmental progress of the child and the relationship is clearly influenced adversely. Indeed, the child may lose previously acquired developmental skills.

11–20 Grossly Impaired

Relationships in this range of functioning are dangerously disorganized. Interactions are disturbed so frequently that the infant is in imminent danger of physical harm.

1–10 Documented maltreatment

The relationship contains documented neglect and physical or sexual abuse that is adversely affecting the child's physical and emotional development.

Relationship Problems Checklist (RPCL)

The clinician should refer to the listing of descriptive features below the scale before using the Relationship Problems Checklist. Each quality of the parent–infant relationship is described in terms of (1) characteristic behavioral quality, (2) affective tone, and (3) psychological involvement. The listed features are not intended to be criteria but guidelines for description. The user should check an appropriate designation for each quality, as indicating "no evidence", "some evidence; needs further investigation", or "substantial evidence."

Relationship Problems Checklist			
Relationship quality	**No evidence**	**Some evidence; needs further investigation**	**Substantial evidence**
Overinvolved	_____	_____	_____
Underinvolved	_____	_____	_____
Anxious/Tense	_____	_____	_____
Angry/Hostile	_____	_____	_____
Verbally Abusive	_____	_____	_____
Physically Abusive	_____	_____	_____
Sexually Abusive	_____	_____	_____

Descriptive Features of Relationship Qualities:

Overinvolved

The relationship is characterized by parental physical and/or psychological overinvolvement that is manifest in the behavioral quality of the interaction, affective tone, and quality of psychological involvement

A. *Behavioral Quality of Interaction*

1. The parent often interferes with the infant or young child's goals and desires.
2. The parent dominates the infant or young child.
3. The parent makes developmentally inappropriate demands.
4. The infant may appear diffuse, unfocused, and undifferentiated.
5. The infant or young child may display submissive, overly compliant behaviors or, conversely, defiant behaviors.
6. In interaction with the parent, the infant or young child may appear to be delayed in motor skills, expressive language, or both.

B. *Affective Tone*

1. The parent may have periods of anxiety, depression, or anger, which result in a lack of consistency in the parent–child interaction.

2. The infant or young child may express anger/obstinacy passively or actively. The infant may whine.

3. The infant or young child's range of affective expression may be very constricted.

C. *Psychological Involvement*

1. The parent may perceive the infant or young child as a partner or peer, or may romanticize or eroticize the child.

2. The parent does not see infant or young child as a separate person with individual needs; the parent is not genuinely interested in the child's uniqueness. Generational boundaries in the family may be diffuse.

3. The infant or young child may cling to the parent and vehemently resist separation.

Underinvolved

The parent may show only sporadic, infrequent involvement or connectedness with the infant or young child. Lack of connectedness is often reflected in the low quality of care offered by the parent directly or purchased as child care.

A. *Behavioral Quality of Interaction*

1. The parent is insensitive and/or unresponsive to the cues of the infant or young child.

2. Consistency is lacking between the parent's expressed attitudes about the infant or young child and the quality of observed interactions. Predictability, reciprocity, or both may be missing from the order and sequence of interactions.

3. The parent ignores, rejects, or fails to comfort the infant or young child.

4. The parent does not adequately mirror the infant or young child's behavior through appropriate reflection of the child's internal feeling states.

5. The parent does not adequately protect the infant or young child from sources of physical or emotional harm, or abuse by others.

6. The parent often misses or misinterprets the infant or young child's cues.

7. The parent and child often appear to be disengaged, with little eye contact or physical proximity.

8. The infant or young child may appear physically and/or psychologically uncared for.

9. Due to a lack of nurturing support for development, the infant or young child may appear delayed in motor and language skills. Some infants, however, may be precocious in motor and language skills, using these capacities as part of a promiscuous character style with adults.

B. Affective Tone

1. Affect in both parent and child is often sad, constricted, withdrawn, and flat.

2. To the observer, the parent–infant or parent–child interaction suggests lifelessness and an absence of pleasure.

C. Psychological Involvement

1. The parent may not demonstrate awareness of the infant or young child's cues or needs in discussions with others or in interactions with the infant.

2. A parent may have experienced emotional deprivation, physical neglect, or both. As a consequence, the parent may be unaware of the infant's needs.

Anxious/Tense

Interactions in this parent–child relationship are tense and constricted, with little sense of relaxed enjoyment or mutuality.

A. Behavioral Quality of Interaction

1. The parent may have a heightened sensitivity to the infant or young child's cues.

2. The parent expresses frequent concern regarding the child's well-being, behavior, or development. To an observer the parent may appear "overprotective."

3. The parent's physical handling of the infant may be awkward or tense.

4. The relationship may involve verbally/emotionally negative interactions, but these are not the primary quality of the relationship.

5. The infant or young child's temperament or developmental capacities do not meet the parent's expectations.

6. The infant or young child may be unusually compliant or anxious around the parent.

B. Affective Tone

1. The parent or child exhibits an anxious mood—as seen in motor tension, apprehension, agitation, facial expressions, and quality of vocalization or speech.

2. Because both parent and infant or young child tend to overreact, they overreact to each other. A pattern of escalating, dysregulating interactions often coexists with underlying regulatory difficulties in the child.

C. Psychological Involvement

The parent who is anxious or tense often misinterprets the child's behavior and/or affect and, consequently, responds inappropriately.

Angry/Hostile

This relationship is characterized by parent–child interactions that are harsh and abrupt, often lacking in emotional reciprocity.

A. Behavioral Quality of the Interaction

1. The parent may be insensitive to the infant's cues, especially when she views the infant as demanding.

2. The parent handles the infant abruptly.

3. The parent may taunt or tease the infant or young child.

4. The infant or young child may appear frightened, anxious, inhibited, impulsive, or diffusely aggressive.

5. The infant or young child may exhibit defiant or resistant behavior with the parent.

6. The infant or young child may exhibit demanding and/or aggressive behaviors with the parent.

7. The infant or young child may exhibit fearful, vigilant, and avoidant behaviors.

8. The infant or young child may show a tendency toward concrete behavior rather than the development of fantasy and imagination. Certain aspects of cognition and language having to do with forming abstractions, as well as coping with complex feelings, may be inhibited or delayed.

B. Affective Tone

1. Interactions between parent and child typically have a hostile or angry edge.

2. An observer is likely to note moderate to considerable tension between the parent and infant or young child, and a noticeable lack of enjoyment or enthusiasm.

3. The infant or young child's affect may be constricted.

C. Psychological Involvement

The parent may view the infant's dependence as demanding and resent the infant's neediness. This resentment may be due to current life stressors or stem from the parent's own relationship history, which may have been characterized by emotional deprivation and/or hostility.

Abusive

Abuse may be verbal, physical, and/or sexual. The three types of abuse described below take precedence, from the point of view of diagnostic classification, over the relationship problems described above. If an abusive pattern applies to the situation, the clinician should use it as the primary relationship diagnosis. The clinician should then characterize the ongoing overall pattern of the relationship, using one of the above relationship descriptions (e.g., underinvolved, angry/tense).

Because of the level of severity and persistence of abusive behaviors, one descriptor from Behavioral Quality of Interaction for any form of abuse is sufficient to determine this classification. Of course, more than one descriptor may apply.

Verbally Abusive

The relationship involves severe abusive emotional content, unclear boundaries, and overcontrol by the parent.

A. Behavioral Quality of the Interaction

1. The content of verbal/emotional abuse by the parent is intended to severely belittle, blame, attack, overcontrol, and/or reject the infant or toddler.

2. The infant or toddler's reactions to verbal/emotional abuse may vary widely, from constriction and vigilance to severe acting-out behaviors. (This variation will depend on the parent's projective contents and the infant's temperament and developmental level.)

B. Affective Tone

1. The negative, abusive nature of the parent–child interaction may be reflected in the infant or young child's depressed, dysregulated, and/or sober affect.

C. Psychological Involvement

1. The parent may misinterpret the infant's cries, often viewing these as deliberate negative reactions toward herself. This misinterpretation may be observed in the verbal content of the parent's attacks, which reflect unresolved issues in previous critical relationships.

2. Signals from the infant may stir up early painful experiences, such as in the case of a mother who cannot bring herself to respond to her

infant's cries because of her own experiences of neglect or who feels inadequate and unworthy when unable to comfort the infant. This connection is often not conscious.

Physically Abusive

The relationship involves severe physical abuse, unclear boundaries, and overcontrol by the parent.

A. Behavioral Quality of Interaction

1. The parent physically harms the infant or child.

2. The parent regularly fails to meet the infant or young child's essential needs for survival, including food, medical care, and/or opportunity to rest.

3. This diagnosis may also include periods of verbal/emotional abuse and/or sexual abuse.

B. Affective Tone

1. The emotional tone of the dyad reflects anger, hostility, or irritability.

2. Considerable to moderate tension and anxiety exist between the parent and infant or young child, with a noticeable lack of enjoyment or enthusiasm.

C. Psychological Involvement

1. The parent exhibits and/or describes anger or hostility toward the infant or young child through abrupt voice or behavior (e.g., scowls, frowns, and exhibits harsh punitive verbal content and/or attitude). The parent shows difficulty setting limits in a non-attacking manner.

2. The infant or young child may evidence a tendency toward concrete behavior rather than the development of fantasy and imagination. Certain aspects of cognition and language having to do with forming abstractions, as well as coping with complex feelings, may be inhibited or delayed.

3. Parent–child interaction may include periods of closeness or enmeshment and of distance, avoidance, or hostility.

4. Parent and infant may function reasonably well in certain areas, but become either too involved or too distant around certain "triggering" issues.

Sexually Abusive

The relationship involves a lack of regard for physical boundaries and extreme sexualized intrusiveness.

A. Behavioral Quality

1. The parent engages in sexually seductive and overstimulating behavior with the infant or young child. The behaviors are intended to gratify the adult's sexual needs or desires.

2. The young child may evidence sexually driven behaviors such as exhibiting himself or trying to look at or touch other children beyond what is developmentally typical.

3. This relationship problem may also include periods of verbal/emotional abuse and/or physical abuse.

B. Affective Tone

1. The lack of boundaries and consistency in parent–infant interaction may be reflected in the parent's affect, which may be labile. Periods of anger or anxiety may be observable.

2. The infant may appear anxious and/or tense.

3. The young child may be fearful, anxious, or diffusely aggressive.

C. Psychological Involvement

1. The parent characteristically fails to respond empathically to the infant or young child's needs and cues, due to preoccupation with his own needs for narcissistic self-gratification.

2. The parent has and may evidence extremely distorted thinking, permitting choice of the young infant as a sexual object.

Axis III

Medical and Developmental Disorders and Conditions

Axis III should be used to note any physical (including medical and neurological), and/or developmental diagnoses made using other diagnostic and classification systems. These systems include the American Psychiatric Association's *Diagnostic and Statistical Manual* (DSM-IV-TR, 2000), *International Classification of Diseases* (ICD-9, 1977, or ICD-10, 1992), and specific classifications used by speech/language pathologists, occupational therapists, physical therapists, special educators, and primary health care providers. If the child meets criteria for a DSM-IV-TR or ICD-10 psychiatric disorder, the disorder should be coded on Axis I as an 800 disorder.

Many psychiatric symptoms can be caused by medical illnesses. Hence, a pediatric or other medical evaluation is highly recommended for many young children who present with psychiatric symptoms. Such an evaluation may also involve clinically indicated developmental and other studies, including laboratory tests. The following examples are illustrative but not exhaustive:

- Infants and young children with symptoms of mood disorder may require a medical evaluation for endocrine disorders. For example, a young child who exhibits lethargy, hypersomnia, low arousability, and poor feeding may need an evaluation for hypothyroidism.

- Infants and young children who have experienced an abrupt onset of irritability, restlessness, and motor dyscoordination may need an evaluation for heavy metal toxicity (e.g., lead, mercury, and manganese).

- Young children who experience an abrupt onset of obsessive or compulsive symptoms should receive a medical evaluation for Pediatric Autoimmune Neuropsychiatric Disorders Associated with Streptococcus (PANDAS). A PANDAS evaluation is particularly important when there is a family history of Obsessive Compulsive Disorder.

- Symptoms of irritability, frustration, and behavioral dysregulation may be a consequence of other conditions that require a hearing test and speech/language evaluation.

Axis IV
Psychosocial Stressors

Axis IV provides a framework for identifying and evaluating psychosocial and environmental stressors that may influence the presentation, course, treatment, and prevention of mental health symptoms and disorders in young children. Specific stressors and, more typically, cumulative stressors during the earliest years of life affect not only the development of disorders but also their likely outcome.

Psychosocial stress in the life of an infant or young child may be acute or enduring. Examples of the latter include poverty, violence in the environment, and abuse in the home. Moreover, stress may be attributable to a single source or it may involve multiple and cumulative events; it may be direct (e.g., an illness requiring a child's hospitalization) or indirect (e.g., a sudden illness of a parent that results in separation from the child).

It is noteworthy that events and transitions that are part of normal experience in the family's culture may nevertheless be stressful for an infant or young child—for example, the birth of a sibling, a family move, a parent returning to work after being at home, or entry into child care or preschool. Some children will experience these transitions as stressful while others make transitions smoothly and adapt to new circumstances easily.

The caregiving environment may shield and protect the child from the stressor, thus lessening its impact; it may compound the impact by failing to offer protection; or it may reinforce the impact of the stressor through the effect of anxiety and/or other negative attitudes.

The ultimate impact of a stressful event or enduring stress depends on three factors:

1. The severity of the stressor (its intensity and duration, the suddenness of the initial stress, and the frequency and unpredictability of its recurrence);
2. The developmental level of the infant or young child (chronological age, social emotional history, biological vulnerability to stress, and ego strength); and

3. The availability and capacity of adults in the caregiving environment to serve as a protective buffer and to help the child understand and cope with the stressor.

The Psychosocial and Environmental Stressor Checklist

The Psychosocial and Environmental Stressor Checklist provides the clinician with a framework for (1) identifying the multiple sources of stress experienced by an individual infant or young child and the family, and (2) noting their duration and severity.

In order to capture the cumulative severity of stressors, the clinician should identify all the sources of stress in a child's circumstances. For example, an infant or young child who enters foster placement may be experiencing the impact of abuse, parental psychiatric illness, separation, and poverty. The greater the number of stressors involved, the greater the adverse impact on the child is presumed to be. When diagnosing Posttraumatic Stress Disorder (Axis I) and Documented Maltreatment (the most disordered relationship category on the PIR-GAS), the clinician should be sure to record the type, onset, and severity of all psychosocial and environmental stressors.

Psychosocial and Environmental Stressor Checklist *(Complete information for all stressors that apply)*		
	Age of onset (in months)	**Comments, including duration and severity**
Challenges to child's primary support group		
Birth of a sibling		
Change in primary caregiver		
Child adopted		
Child in foster care		
Child in institutional care		
Death of a parent		
Death of other family member		
Death of nonfamily significant other		
Domestic violence		
Emotional abuse		
Marital discord		
Medical illness of parent (specify acute or chronic)		

Psychosocial and Environmental Stressor Checklist *(continued)*	Age of onset (in months)	Comments, including duration and severity
Medical illness of sibling (specify acute or chronic)		
Neglect		
New adult in household (e.g., boyfriend)		
New child (not by birth) in home (e.g. adoption, stepsibling, cousin)		
Parental divorce or separation		
Parental mental illness		
Parental remarriage		
Parental separation from child (e.g., out-of-town employment, hospitalization)		
Parental separation (work)		
Parental substance abuse		
Physical abuse		
Removal of child from home		
Severe discord or violence with sibling		
Sexual abuse		
Sibling mental illness		
Sibling substance abuse		
Challenges in the social environment		
Cultural conflicts		
Discrimination		
Inadequate social support for the family		
Single parenting		
Educational/child care challenges		
More than 9 hours/day in out-of-home care		
Multiple changes in child care provider		
Parent without high school diploma		
Parental illiteracy or low literacy		
Poor-quality early learning environment (e.g., health and safety concerns; high child/ staff ratios and large groups; inadequately trained staff; lack of attention to social and emotional development)		

Psychosocial and Environmental Stressor Checklist *(continued)*	Age of onset (in months)	Comments, including duration and severity
Housing challenges		
Dislocation from home		
Homelessness		
Multiple moves		
Problems maintaining heat, electricity, water, and telephone		
Unsafe neighborhood		
Unsafe or overcrowded housing		
Economic challenges		
Food insecurity		
Heavy indebtedness		
Poverty or near poverty		
Occupational challenges		
Dangerous or stressful parental work conditions (civilian)		
Military deployment		
Parental unemployment		
Threat of parental job loss		
Health-care access challenges		
Inadequate health services in area		
Lack of or inadequate health insurance		
Health of child		
Hospitalization of child		
Medical illness in child (acute or chronic); child accident/injury (e.g. animal bite, passenger in vehicular accident)		
Medical procedure(s) performed on child (e.g., spinal tap)		
Legal/criminal justice challenges		
Child Protective Services involvement		
Child victim of crime		
Custody dispute in the context of parental divorce		
Immigration status		

Psychosocial and Environmental Stressor Checklist *(continued)*		
	Age of onset (in months)	**Comments, including duration and severity**
Parental arrest		
Parental incarceration		
Parent victim of crime		
Other		
Abduction (specify by family member or nonfamily member)		
Child witness to violence (in the home)		
Child witness to violence (out of the home)		
Epidemic (e.g., AIDS)		
Natural disaster (e.g., fire, hurricane)		
War/terrorism		
Other		
Other		

Axis V
Emotional and Social Functioning

Axis V reflects the infant or young child's emotional and social functioning in the context of interaction with important caregivers and in relation to expectable patterns of development in the earliest years.

Emotional and social capacities are present at birth. As newborns adapt to sensations outside the womb, they exhibit significant individual differences in their capacities to self-regulate their states of arousal and their emotions. Infants and young children also differ in their ability to interact socially with those in the caregiving environment. As infants and young children develop physically and neurologically, their capacities to regulate and interact socially also progress. The child makes use of earlier capacities to reach higher levels of functioning. In this process, new capacities emerge.

Rating Capacities for Emotional and Social Functioning

A number of capacities contribute to a young child's emotional and social functioning. (See below for definitions and the ages at which the capacities are likely to be observable in typically developing children.) Six of these capacities include:

1. Attention and regulation;
2. Forming relationships or mutual engagement;
3. Intentional two-way communication;
4. Complex gestures and problem solving;
5. Use of symbols to express thoughts and feelings; and
6. Connecting symbols logically and abstract thinking.

In the course of an assessment, it is appropriate for the clinician to observe the quality of the infant or young child's play and interaction with *each* of the significant people in her life. The clinician should then choose the rating that best fits the child's functioning with respect to each of the capacities listed above in interaction with each caregiver.

For each of the capacities, the clinician may report that the child:

1. Functions at an age-appropriate level under all conditions and with a full range of affect states.

2. Functions at an age-appropriate level, but is vulnerable to stress or with a constricted range of affect or both.

3. Functions immaturely (i.e., has the capacity, but not at an age-appropriate level).

4. Functions inconsistently or intermittently unless special structure or sensorimotor support is available.

5. Barely evidences this capacity, even with support.

6. Has not achieved this capacity.

The clinician should use a rating of "not applicable" (n/a) when the child is below the age at which he would typically be expected to have the capacity in question.

Capacities for Emotional and Social Functioning Rating Scale

The Capacities for Emotional and Social Functioning Rating Scale can be used to create a summary of the child's overall pattern of emotional and social functioning. Because documenting best performance is important for intervention

Capacities for Emotional and Social Functioning Rating Scale							
Emotional and social functioning capacities	**Functional rating**						
	1.	**2.**	**3.**	**4.**	**5.**	**6.**	**n/a**
Attention and regulation							
Forming relationships/mutual engagement							
Intentional two-way communication							
Complex gestures and problem solving							
Use of symbols to express thoughts/feelings							
Connecting symbols logically/abstract thinking							

planning, the summary should describe the child's highest level of functioning. The summary should also report inconsistencies in functioning.

Description of Capacities for Emotional and Social Functioning

The six capacities for emotional and social functioning that are described below correspond to the functional emotional developmental levels listed in DC:0–3, but we have modified some of the terminology.

- **Attention and regulation** (typically observable beginning between birth and 3 months)—The infant notices and attends to what is going on in the world through all the senses—for example, by looking, listening, touching, and moving. The infant can stay sufficiently regulated to attend and interact, without over- or underreacting to external or internal stimuli. As the child achieves higher levels of functioning over time, her capacity to maintain a long, continuous flow of interactions provides evidence of her capacity for age-appropriate attention and regulation.

- **Forming relationships or mutual engagement** (typically observable beginning between 3 and 6 months)—The infant develops a relationship with an emotionally available caregiver for soothing, security, and pleasure. As development proceeds, with support from the caregiving environment, the child becomes able to experience the full range of positive and negative emotions while remaining engaged in a relationship.

- **Intentional two-way communication** (typically observable beginning between 4 and 10 months)—The infant uses gestures, including purposeful demonstrations of affect, to start reciprocal "conversations." Simple gestures, such as reaching to be picked up or pointing to an object of interest, become a more complex sequence of gestures during the second year. Two-way communication becomes actual conversation as the child develops verbal language,

- **Complex gestures and problem solving** (typically observable beginning between 10 and 18 months)—The toddler learns how to use emerging motor skills and language to get what he needs or wants—that is, to solve problems. Single gestures are replaced by complex sequences of gestures and actions (e.g., leading a parent to a desired object). As the child develops language, he uses words as well as gestures for communication and problem solving.

- **Use of symbols to express thoughts and feelings** (typically observable beginning between 18 and 30 months)—Using imaginative play and language, the child begins to express thoughts, ideas, and feelings through symbols. A child can communicate what she imagines through role-play, dress-up, and play with dolls and action figures. Imaginative play may represent experiences from real life, as well as themes the child has encountered in stories, books, videos, and television. In her play scenarios, the child projects her own feelings onto the characters and actions.

- **Connecting symbols logically and abstract thinking** (typically observable beginning between 30 and 48 months)—The child can connect and elaborate sequences of ideas logically. He uses logically interconnected ideas in conversations about daily events and imaginative stories. The narratives of children who function at this level typically have a beginning, middle, and end. They include characters with clear motives and consequences of action that can be anticipated. The child is able to understand abstract concepts, reflect on feelings, and articulate lessons that he has learned from an experience.

In children who are developing typically, each of these six core capacities continues to develop as the child matures. Each fully mastered ability supports progress toward the next level of development within that capacity (e.g., competent gestural communication supports the development of spoken language). Some children, however, may show a constricted form of a higher-level capacity without having fully achieved more basic levels of emotional and social functioning. For example, a preschooler may express many ideas in self-absorbed play but remain unable to attend and engage interactively, even at the level that one would expect to see in a much younger child.

Appendix A
Prioritizing Diagnostic Classification and Planning Intervention

Clinical formulation results from a diagnostic process in which the clinician or team draws together multiple observations and sources of information about an individual child within a general diagnostic scheme. Proper use of the DC:0–3R for clinical formulation requires that the clinician document and analyze observations and ratings on all five axes of DC:0–3R with an outcome that includes a coherent plan for what the clinician should do next to assist the child and family. This section provides guidelines for prioritizing diagnostic classification on Axis I and identifying a primary diagnosis for purposes of intervention.

Prioritizing Diagnostic Classification

DC:0–3R recognizes that for some infants and young children, more than one diagnostic classification may be appropriate. The clinician's job is to list all the diagnostic classifications for which the child's symptoms and other circumstances meet criteria. Moreover, some maladaptive behaviors of infants and young children (e.g., somatic symptoms, irritability, withdrawal, impulsivity, fears, and developmental delays) appear in more than one of the clinical disorders in Axis I. Because an infant or young child can respond to stress in only a limited number of ways, some overlap of behavioral patterns is inevitable. Thus, comorbidity between disorders is allowed in DC:0–3R. Nonetheless, it is clinically helpful to prioritize diagnoses and identify the primary diagnosis that will be the initial target of the intervention.

Wright and Northcutt (2004) have advanced a "decision tree" guideline for prioritizing diagnostic classification under DC:0–3. They are preparing a DC:0–3R version. We anticipate that a DC:0–3R version will also be proposed.

Choosing a Primary Diagnostic Category

These guidelines are designed to help the clinician decide which diagnostic category to designate as primary for a given set of difficulties.

1. If there is a clear stress condition that is significant and is associated with the disordered behavior or emotions (e.g., a specific overwhelming episode or multiple repeated traumatic events), consider Posttraumatic Stress Disorder as a primary diagnosis.

2. If a child has lost a primary caregiver and symptoms meet criteria for Bereavement Disorder, give Bereavement Disorder precedence as the primary diagnosis, above other diagnostic classifications.

3. If a clear constitutionally or individually based sensory, motor, processing, organizational, or integration difficulty is associated with the observed maladaptive behavioral and/or emotional patterns (regardless of the particular symptoms), consider Regulation Disorders of Sensory Processing. Clinical experience with this diagnostic classification suggests the possibility of co-occurrences (co-morbidity) with other Axis I categories.

4. If presenting problems are mild, of less than 4 months' duration, and associated with a clear environmental event, such as a parent's return to work, a move, or change in child care, consider an Adjustment Disorder diagnosis.

5. Without a clear constitutionally or individually based vulnerability or a severe or significant stress or trauma, and when the difficulty is not mild, of short duration, or associated with a clear event, consider the categories of Disorders of Affect.

6. Disorders of Communication and Social Relatedness are extreme and distinct enough to be recognizable in their own right. They usually involve chronic patterns of maladaptation and multiple areas of delay. These disorders should take precedence over other categories such as Regulatory Disorders of Sensory Processing or Posttraumatic Stress Disorder. However, co-occurring diagnoses may be considered when warranted (for example, in response to a trauma).

7. If the child's only difficulty involves a caring or parental relationship, and there are no other symptoms independent of that relationship, use Axis II: Relationship Classification rather than Axis I: Clinical Disorders to indicate the nature of the difficulty. An Axis II classification may be appropriate, for example, for a child who is depressed only in the child care setting or a child who is very labile emotionally only in the presence of a particular caregiver.

8. When a child experiences difficulty only in a certain situation or in relation to a particular person, consider the diagnoses of Adjustment Disorder or Relationship Disorder.

9. Reserve the designation of Deprivation/Maltreatment Disorder to describe seriously inadequate physical, psychological, and emotional care. Use Axis II: Relationship Classification to record other concerns about a caregiving relationship.

10. When common symptoms such as feeding and sleep behavior disorders are present, assess the underlying basis for these difficulties, which may be problems in their own right or part of other diagnostic categories. For example, feeding or eating difficulties may begin following an acute trauma, represent a temporary reaction to a stressful change (such as a move or to a parent's going to work), or be related to physical problems. These difficulties may also be part of an ongoing pattern, as in a Deprivation/Maltreatment Disorder, a Regulation Disorder of Sensory Processing, or a Disorder of Relating and Communicating. They may also occur as part of a pattern in a Relationship Disorder (Axis II).

11. DC:0–3 guidelines encouraged clinicians to choose a single diagnostic classification wherever possible. DC:0–3R, drawing upon more than 10 years of clinical experience, indicates that more than one primary diagnostic classification on Axis I may often be appropriate. Thus, a Sleep Behavior Disorder and a Separation Anxiety Disorder may co-occur, as well as a Regulatory Disorder of Sensory Processing and Depression. In such instances, it may be appropriate to highlight two primary diagnoses for purposes of treatment planning. In any case, all diagnoses that meet specified criteria should be listed in any given clinical formulation.

The Process of Revising DC:0–3

Revising DC:0–3

A 2-year plan for carrying out the revision was presented to the Executive Committee of ZERO TO THREE in December 2002 and approved in January 2003. The plan included: a survey of users of DC:0–3; a review of clinical literature; drafting a preliminary version of minor revisions to DC:0–3; a second user survey to elicit comments on the preliminary minor revisions; and additional communications with clinical experts in specific areas of diagnosis and treatment. The plan also included connecting with work that was being completed at the time, sponsored by the American Academy of Child and Adolescent Psychiatry, for extending DSM-IV criteria into the preschool age period with research diagnostic criteria (see RDC-PA, 2003). A 2-year schedule was considered important for progress to occur with a needed revision of DC:0–3, recognizing that the resulting guide would be imperfect but could then contribute to subsequent clinical trials and research. A timely revision, in other words, could facilitate continuing evolution of the diagnostic system so that a later major revision would be possible.

Accordingly, a revision task group was formed whose members worked both independently and collaboratively and conferred regularly via conference calls, e-mail, and face-to-face meetings throughout the 2-year period. Members of the work group were Helen Egger, Emily Fenichel, Antoine Guedeney, Brian Wise, Harry Wright, and Robert Emde (chair). Margaret Henry and Crystal Wiggins served as staff assistants. Helen Egger and Harry Wright had served on the independent RDC-PA task force; Robert Emde, who presented the original plan for the revision to ZERO TO THREE, had served on the original task force that developed DC:0–3. Members of the revision task force had training in child and adolescent psychiatry, epidemiology, general psychiatry, and social work. Two clinical psychologists who were invited to join the work group were unable to do so.

Results of an Initial Users' Survey

In June 2003 the work group conducted a Web-based survey of 1200 users of DC:0–3. E-mail invitations with links to the survey instrument were sent to all users for whom we had access, including participants in DC:0–3 training sessions; all members of the World Association for Infant Mental Health and the German Association for Infant Mental Health; experts in the assessment of infants and young children identified by the National Institute of Mental Health; ZERO TO THREE Board Members, Fellows and staff; and other groups of senior infant and early childhood mental health clinicians. The survey instrument included multiple-choice and open-ended questions dealing with areas of professional discipline, and practice (including usual diagnostic procedures), experience with DC:0–3, as well as opinions about its usefulness.

Two hundred forty-five individuals from 24 countries (62% from the United States) responded to the survey. Respondents identified themselves, in order of frequency, as infant mental health specialists, clinical psychologists, child psychiatrists, parent–infant specialists, social workers, special educators, psychoanalysts, program administrators, and occupational therapists. Respondents were quite experienced in clinical work with children from birth to age 5. Two thirds had more than 10 years' experience; only 14% had less than 5 years' experience. We asked respondents to list the five most frequent mental health disorders they saw in the 0–5 age group; the most frequently mentioned were, in order: Regulatory Disorders, Disorders of Relating and Communicating, disruptive behaviors, Anxiety Disorders, Reactive Attachment Disorder, Posttraumatic Stress Disorder, Feeding Behavior Disorders, Sleep Behavior Disorders, and depression.

Of the respondents, 50% said they used DC:0–3 frequently, most of the time, or always in making assessments. Nine percent of respondents said they were either not currently using DC:0–3 or had never used the system. Respondents identified the following DC:0–3 Axis I classification categories as especially useful: Disorders of Relating and Communicating, Regulatory Disorders, Traumatic Stress Disorder, Reactive Attachment Deprivation/ Maltreatment Disorder, and Adjustment Disorder. A significant number of respondents mentioned these categories as not useful: Gender Identity Disorder, Mixed Disorder of Emotional Expressiveness, Depression of Infancy and Early Childhood, Sleep Behavior Disorders, and Reactive Attachment Deprivation/Maltreatment Disorder. Approximately one half of respondents said they used Axis II: Relationship Disorders frequently, most of the time, or always; an equal number said they used Axis II seldom or never. The majority of respondents found Axes III–V useful.

To questions about their diagnostic practices, 69% of respondents answered that they routinely used three sessions or more for diagnostic assessment of infants, toddlers, and young children; 40% said they used four or more sessions. Sources of information for more than 75% of respondents included parent/family reports, clinician interactions with the child, general clinical impressions, and observation of parent–child play.

Prompted by open-ended questions, respondents identified sections of DC:0–3 that needed clarification, pointed out gaps in criteria, and suggested changes in wording. More generally, they wrote of the need to incorporate new knowledge and research into diagnostic criteria that could, in turn, improve the usefulness of the system.

Drafting, a Second Survey, and Further Input

Work group members systematically reviewed survey results and reviewed all literature relevant to mental health disorders of infancy and early childhood. As we began to develop diagnostic criteria in biweekly conference calls, we paid close attention to the Research Diagnostic Criteria–Preschool Age classification system (RDC-PA). Despite the RDC–PA's focus on the post-infancy years, wherever possible, we wanted to connect with these criteria, for two reasons: (1) consistency—they represented the consensus of a previous task force on criteria that were linked to evidence—and (2) descriptive specificity—criteria reflected enough detail that reliability could be meaningfully assessed.

In December 2003, we completed a preliminary version of DC:0–3R, presenting major aspects of it at the World Association of Infant Mental Health Congress in Melbourne, Australia, in January 2004. Guided by feedback from the international group of participants at the Congress, we circulated a second draft to the 80% of initial survey respondents who had indicated their willingness to review a draft DC:0–3R. On the basis of the responses to this query, we gathered specific suggestions about wording of criteria.

During the second half of 2004, the work group concentrated on seeking comments from individuals and groups of clinical researchers who were working in areas where we had found substantial differences of opinion among clinicians and researchers. These areas included Regulatory Disorders of Sensory Processing, Disorders of Relating and Communicating, Posttraumatic Stress Disorder, and Deprivation/Maltreatment Disorder. Additional revisions resulted in a penultimate version of DC:0–3R, which was sent for final review to a panel of expert infant mental health clinicians for review and final comments.

Diagnostic Classification of Mental Health and Developmental Disorders of Infancy and Early Childhood Revised Edition (DC:0–3R) is the result of the 2-year process that we have described.

Appendix C
ZERO TO THREE Diagnostic Classification Task Force

Developers of the original *Diagnostic Classification of Mental Health and Developmental Disorders of Infancy and Early Childhood (DC:0–3),* published in 1994, were:

Members

Stanley Greenspan, MD, Chair

Serena Wieder, PhD, Co-Chair

Kathryn Barnard, RN, PhD

Irene Chatoor, MD

Roseanne Clark, PhD

Robert N. Emde, MD

Robert J. Harmon, MD

Alicia F. Lieberman, PhD

Reginald Lourie, MD

Klaus Minde, MD

Joy D. Osofsky, PhD

Sally Provence, MD

Chaya Roth, PhD

Bertram Ruttenberg, MD

Arnold Sameroff, PhD

Rebecca Shahmoon-Shanok, MSW, PhD

Albert J. Solnit, MD

Charles Zeanah, MD

Barry Zuckerman, MD

Mark Applebaum, PhD, Research Consultant

Participants, Phase II

Clara Aisenstein, PhD

Marie Anzalone, SciD

Stephen Bennett, MD

Susan Berger, PhD

Barbara Dunbar, PhD

Marguerite Dunitz, MD

Alice Frankel, MD

Eva Gochman, PhD

Peter Gorski, MD

Joyce Hopkins, PhD

Peter Scheer, MD

Madeline Shalowitz, MD

Jean Thomas, MSW, MD

Sylvia Turner, MD

Donna Weston, PhD

Carol Wheeler-Liston, PhD

Molly Romer Witten, PhD

References

American Psychiatric Association. (2000). *Diagnostic and statistical manual of mental disorders (DSM-IV-TR),* (4th ed., text revision). Washington, DC: Author.

American Psychiatric Association. (1994). *Diagnostic and statistical manual of mental disorders (DSM-IV),* (4th ed.,). Washington, DC: Author.

American Psychiatric Association. (1987). *Diagnostic and statistical manual of mental disorders (DSM-III-R),* (3rd ed., revised). Washington, DC: Author.

Emde, R. N., & Wise, B. K. (2003). The cup is half full: Initial clinical trials of DC:0–3 and a recommendation for revision. *Infant Mental Health Journal, 24*(4), 437–446.

Guedeney, A., & Maestro, S. (Eds.). (2003). The use of the Diagnostic Classification 0–3. [Special Issue]. *Infant Mental Health Journal, 24*(3).

Task Force on Research Diagnostic Criteria: Infancy and Preschool. (2003). Research diagnostic criteria for infants and preschool children: The process and empirical support. *Journal of the American Academy of Child & Adolescent Psychiatry, 42*(12), 1504–1512. Further information available at www.infantinstitute.org.

World Health Organization. (1977). *International classification of diseases, 9th revision.* Geneva, Switzerland: Author.

World Health Organization. (1992). *International statistical classification of diseases and related health problems, 10th revision.* Geneva, Switzerland: Author.

Wright, C., & Northcutt, C. (2004). Schematic decision trees for DC:0–3. *Infant Mental Health Journal, 25*(3), 171–174.